W9-BYL-164

TAKING CARE OF YOUR NEW BABY

A Guide to Infant Care

Jeanne Driscoll, RN
&
Marsha Walker, RN

 AVERY PUBLISHING GROUP INC.

Garden City Park, New York

Cover Design: Rudy Shur and Martin Hochberg
Cover Photograph: Michel Tcherevkoff Studio, N.Y., N.Y.
Original Illustrations: Vicki Hudon
In-House Editor: Karen Price Heffernan

Library of Congress Cataloging-in-Publication Data

Driscoll, Jeanne Watson.
    Taking care of your new baby : a guide to infant care / Jeanne
Watson Driscoll, Marsha Walker.
        p. cm.
    Bibliography: p.
    Includes index.
    ISBN 0-89529-397-8 : $6.95
    1. Infants (Newborn)—Care—Popular works. 2. Infants
(Newborn)—Health and hygiene—Popular works. I. Walker,
Marsha. II. Title.
RJ253.D75   1989
649'.122—dc20

                              89-6536
                              CIP

Copyright © 1989 by Jeanne Watson Driscoll and Marsha Walker

All rights reserved. No part of this publication may be
reproduced, stored in a retrieval system, or transmitted, in any
form or by any means, electronic, mechanical, photocopying,
recording, or otherwise, without the prior written permission of
the copyright owner.

Printed in the United States of America

10 9 8 7 6 5 4

Contents

Preface

Welcome to parenthood—the most wonderful, challenging, and competitive job in your life! You may or may not have had your baby yet, but one thing you have probably discovered is that everyone else knows how to take care of your baby, whether or not they have children of their own! Babies cause grownups to forget all about social etiquette, and they leave parents wide open for attacks from people who offer hints, tips, and opinions.

Wait until you go to the market and have all the grandmothers there advise you about when the baby should be taken out of the house. Who cares that the only things left in your freezer are ice cubes! "You should be *home* with a baby that small" is the comment of the day.

As you experience parenthood, you will wonder how you ever made it to your age and how you will ever make it as a parent when everyone knows so much more than you do. Well, hang on and welcome to the gang.

Our goal in this book is to share the secrets and give suggestions on how to make the first few weeks at home with a new baby a little easier. We will talk about infant care, common concerns parents have, and the very normal emotional adjustment of Mommy, Daddy, and Baby. We hope that by reading this book you will recognize and accept the feelings of fear, panic, sadness, and joy that you will have; that you will see that you are not alone; and that you will develop a sense of humor (most important!) so that you can laugh at yourself and at the crazy things you will do, think, and say over the next few weeks as you begin to live the course: Parenthood 101.

This course does not come with a syllabus and required reading list. It is learned on the job, by trial and error. The only prerequisite is a baby. The course is based on subjective reality. No two human beings are alike—each is unique and special. On this basis, *there are no rules, only guidelines.*

In other words, what worked for one person or baby may not work with *your* baby. You will be given many suggestions, but *you* must decide what works best for you. In fact, that is one of the first lessons you will learn: smile, accept the advice, thank the giver, sort out the information, and then do what *you* want to do.

Chapter One
Physical Characteristics of Baby

The first time you see your baby is quite an overwhelming experience. After learning whether they have a girl or boy, the next question most parents have is usually "Is he (or she) all right?" Parents are often quite captivated by this new little person and can't take their eyes off him.

However, not all mothers feel instant love. Labor and delivery is an emotional and physically draining experience, and some mothers need to regroup before they can reach out and embrace their newborn. The hospital or alternative birthing center is still not your home. The short time you spend there serves as a brief introduction to your baby, but at home you will have many years to get to know him.

Before you left the hospital, you may have been given loads of information, so some of this may be a review. But you may not remember one word of what was said because you were still in shock with the realization that you actually had a baby and all was well. Some mothers describe this as a time when they were so tired that one thing blended into another and they weren't completely aware of what was happening around them. Mothers also express confusion at all the conflicting advice they hear during their hospital stay. The first concern that most new parents have immediately after delivery is the health of their baby; the second is the appearance of the baby. The following section will discuss how the baby's body will appear, how to care for it, and how it will change.

Have you noticed that your newborn does not look like the babies in magazines and on television? Those babies are usually about three or four months old. Usually, a newborn looks like she has no neck and a head that is too big for her body. Her trunk is long, and her arms and legs appear short because she likes them flexed, as she was *in utero*. Her hands are tightly clenched and her abdomen is big, with sloping shoulders and a round chest. She has miniature toes, with lint between them. If your baby was breech, her feet and legs are probably still flexed up toward her head and she may take several weeks to assume the typical newborn posture. A healthy baby is described in Figure 1.1.

HEAD

Does your child have a "cone head?" Don't be alarmed! This shape is common in a vaginally delivered baby. The molding of the head is due to baby's soft cranial bones, which are designed to conform to the shape of the mother's bony pelvis during the trip down the birth canal. After about two days or so, the head will round out. If you experienced a Cesarean delivery and did not do any pushing, your baby's head is probably nice and round.

The bones that make up the baby's head are not totally joined, which allows the baby's head to mold and also permits space for brain growth. You have probably discovered where these bones have not yet joined. These areas are called **fontanelles,** or soft spots. There are two fontanelles that you may have noticed. The one in the front of the head is the **anterior fontanelle**, three to four centimeters long by two to three centimeters wide. It is covered by a tough membrane and will close by eighteen to twenty-four months. The one in the back of the baby's head is called the **posterior fontanelle**. It is smaller and will close by eight to twelve weeks.

Most parents are concerned about these soft spots. "If I touch them, will I damage her brain?" No! You will not damage the fontanelle or brain with normal handling. In some babies who do not have much hair, you may see a pulse beating under the membrane. This is normal.

Fontanelles ("Soft Spots")
1) Front–diamond shaped
2) Back–triangle shaped

Eyes are slate colored, puffy, with no tears, and may wander. They "see" light and dark, and may be able to distinguish shapes.

Nose is wide and flat. Sense of smell is acute.

Mouth sucks continually. Taste is acute.

Chin is receded.

Hands–The fists are tightly clenched and baby will have long nails.

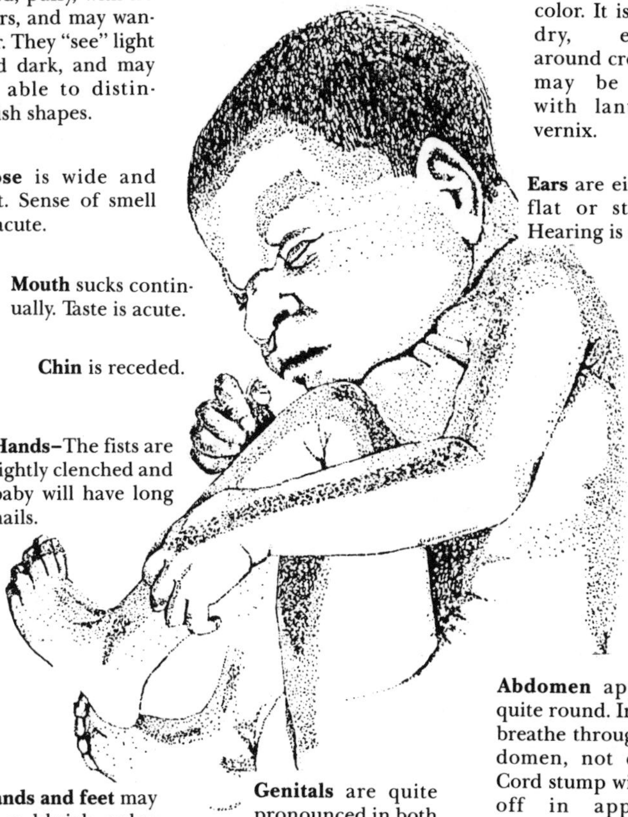

Hands and feet may be a bluish color and cold to the touch.

Feet and Legs are drawn up–returning to fetal position.

Head is generally large in comparison to rest of body (13"–14" in circumference).

Genitals are quite pronounced in both sexes.

Milia–white spots over nose and under eyes.

Average Length
Boys–20"
Girls–19"

Average Weight
Boys–7½ lbs.
Girls–7 lbs.

Skin is ruddy red color. It is thin and dry, especially around creases, and may be covered with lanugo and vernix.

Ears are either very flat or stick out. Hearing is acute.

Abdomen appears quite round. Infants breathe through abdomen, not chest. Cord stump will fall off in approximately 10 days.

Figure 1.1. What a Healthy Newborn Looks Like

Hair and Scalp

Your baby may have been born with an incredible amount of thick hair or he may look like a cue ball, with almost no hair at all. Much of the newborn hair may fall out and be replaced with new hair that may or may not be the color of the hair he was born with.

In the early days or weeks you may be admiring your baby's hair and suddenly discover yellowish crusty patches on his scalp. Oh no! The dread condition called **cradle cap**! We hope that your self-image as parents is not dependent on whether or not your baby has cradle cap! All humans secrete oils from the glands in the scalp. Babies also have skin on the scalp that normally dries and flakes off. Dust and dirt are also present on the scalp and hair. You can wash the hair anywhere from two times a week to every day. Remember—*no rules*!

As for cradle cap—this is a time in your baby's life when his scalp will be secreting increased amounts of oil because of extra hormonal stimulation. This oil can accumulate and dry in patches all over the scalp. It doesn't bother the baby, but it does bother the baby's parents and grandparents.

When you wash baby's hair, massage the scalp to promote circulation and remove oils and dry skin. A soft toothbrush is a wonderful tool to use. You can massage the soft spots and not have to worry about scratching the baby's head with your fingernails.

Cradle cap will gradually resolve by itself. Do not pick at it. Some people recommend softening the crusts with baby oil and then washing it out. Did you ever try washing oil out of your hair? Shampoo hair with baby shampoo or any shampoo or soap that is mild and has no deodorants. Be sure to rinse the scalp well to remove the soap.

If you are worried about how the baby's grandparents will react to this cradle cap, put a bonnet or cap on baby when they come over. Tell them it is to help keep him warm. Who needs to hear criticism of something that is an act of nature!

Eyes

Your baby's eyes may still be a bit puffy or swollen when he arrives home. This puffiness may be from the silver nitrate drops put into his eyes after birth. Some babies have erythromycin or tetracycline ointment put in their eyes, which seems to decrease the irritation. Puffy and bloodshot eyes can also come from the pressures experienced during the process of birth.

Babies do keep their eyes closed in the early days. If you think about it, the baby lived in darkness for forty weeks or so. He is born under bright lights, into a world where grownups make weird faces and speak in octaves three times above normal! No wonder babies keep their eyes closed!

Your baby can see your face quite well right from birth when held at feeding distance (six to ten inches). He does not have distant vision yet, and may not concentrate on your face for very long. Babies can only handle small doses of stimulation before they have to close their eyes and regroup. They are not bored! Try lowering the lights and approaching your baby from the side to look at him. Whisper, then talk a bit louder. Remember, this is all new for this special little baby.

The color of your baby's eyes may be blue, slate blue, or gray. Darker-skinned babies may have eyes with muddy or brown coloring. Eye color is established by about three months, but may change up to one year.

Your baby's eyes may be crossed or seem to wander at times. This is caused by poor control of the muscles around the eyes, and will usually correct itself as the muscles strengthen in about three or four months.

You may or may not notice tears when your baby cries. Some babies do not produce tears until they are two months old. Other babies may have a blocked tear duct so that the eye seems to be filled with tears. Ask your pediatrician any questions you have about your baby's eyes.

Nose

Does your baby sneeze a lot? All babies do. No, she does not have a cold. Her nose is doing what is designed to do—clean the air that she will breathe. If an irritating particle should enter her nose, she will sneeze. Just remove the mucus with a soft diaper, tissue, or washcloth.

Babies are also nose breathers. They do not breathe through their mouth yet. Always make sure that your baby has a clear way for air to get to the nose. Many babies also accumulate enough mucus in the nose to cause them to sneeze or for you to hear sniffles and noises when they breathe.

Have you noticed some "whiteheads" around your baby's nose and chin? These are called **milia**. This is a common newborn skin condition that is a result of unopened (plugged) sebaceous (oil secreting) glands. There is no special treatment for milia. In time, it will go away. These whiteheads should not be squeezed, nor should any preparations be put on them. They will disappear in a few weeks by themselves.

Mouth

Your baby's mouth is an extremely sensitive area. Much of the information about the outside world enters through the mouth. Many of a newborn baby's functions are controlled by reflexes. One of the reflexes of the mouth is called the **rooting reflex**. (See Figure 1.2.) When the side of your baby's mouth or cheek is touched, she will turn toward that side and open her lips and mouth to suck. Premature babies often do not exhibit this rooting reflex until they are a little older. Rooting, sucking, and swallowing reflexes aid baby in feeding.

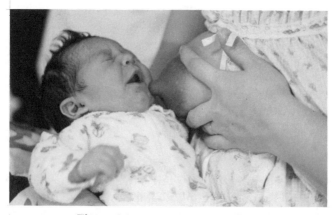

Figure 1.2. The Rooting Reflex

When you breast- or bottle feed your baby, stroke the lower lip or side of her mouth first to help her locate her food. Most babies are born with sucking and rooting reflexes—some just can't get it all together at first when they start eating. The rooting reflex disappears by about seven months of age.

Sucking is important to your baby during the entire first year of life and sometimes beyond. If you feel that your baby seems to be sucking on her fist, your finger, the blanket, and (good grief!) a pacifier, it is because of this need for sucking. Some babies have a stronger need than others. We will talk more about pacifiers (that dirty word!) later.

Some parents think that they can tell if a baby is hungry by testing to see if she will suck on a nipple, breast, or finger. Babies will suck on anything, anytime, even right after a feeding. Please do not use sucking as a test to see if baby should be fed or is getting enough milk.

While you watch your baby cry, you may notice that her tongue is white all over. This is from milk feedings. If, however, you notice white patches that may look like milk curds sticking to the tongue, gums, or insides of your baby's cheeks, this may be a condition called **thrush**. If you try to remove these white patches it may cause some bleeding. Do not worry about this. It is a fungus (called *Candida albicans*), often acquired from Mom's vaginal tract during birth. It is easily treated after you have talked with your pediatrician, and usually disappears quickly with medication, although sometimes it can persist for months. Thrush can also give breastfeeding mothers sore nipples. Ask your doctor how to treat this. Your doctor may prescribe medication for your nipples and your baby's mouth.

You may notice a blister on baby's upper lip. This is a sucking blister, the result of baby's sucking on a nipple. This can appear anytime while baby is still being breast- or bottle fed. Sometimes these blisters disappear between feedings. They do not cause discomfort in baby, and you don't need to worry about them.

SKIN

Many parents are concerned about the appearance of their baby's skin. Your baby's skin color has probably gone through a few changes since birth—from dusky red to mottled with bluish hands and feet. As his circulation becomes more efficient, you will see more normal skin tones. It takes a little while for the circulatory system to become efficient at getting blood around to the extremities.

Jaundice

Now that you are aware of the rainbow of skin colors available to a newborn, let's talk about the color yellow. Newborn babies frequently exhibit what is called **physiologic** or **newborn jaundice**. Most parents are frightened when they are told that their baby has this condition, and an awareness of what this is and what to expect really helps.

Jaundice is not a disease. Instead, it is a symptom of an imbalance in the inner workings of the body. Babies are born with an extra amount of red blood cells. These are necessary during prenatal life to help carry oxygen in the low-oxygen environment of the uterus. Once the baby is born, these excess red blood cells are no longer needed, and break down. One of the waste products released from the cells is a substance called **bilirubin**. Bilirubin is then cleared from the blood by the liver and changed to a form that the baby can excrete. Sometimes, however, the liver may be a little immature to handle this job, so the bilirubin is recirculated, and turns the skin and whites of the eyes yellow! With physiologic jaundice (there are other types), the yellow color usually appears at two or three days of age. The appearance of jaundice before this time or at birth is a cause for more concern as it is not a normal occurrence.

Jaundice may first be noticed while you are still in the hospital, but with early hospital discharges this condition may not appear until after you arrive home. Normal values for an adult are 1mg/dl (mg = milligram; dl = deciliter). Bilirubin can rise to a peak of 7 to 12 mg/dl by the second or third day, and sometimes continues to about 15 mg/dl before it starts back down. Usually nothing needs to be done and this will resolve by itself. Sometimes parents are instructed to undress baby and place him in a window where indirect light can break down the bilirubin (not direct sunlight—we're not growing corn!). Sometimes extra water is given to baby to help him excrete bilirubin. This practice has never been proven to prevent or resolve this condition.

Special phototherapy lights can also be used to drop the bilirubin level faster if it continues to rise or rises suddenly. Babies undergoing phototherapy may be sleepy and not interested in feedings.

You may also have heard of another variation of jaundice called **breast milk jaundice**. This is thought to occur because a factor in the mother's milk inhibits a liver enzyme from doing its job of breaking down bilirubin. There are several other theories about this situation, none of which have yet been shown to be the actual cause. This type of jaundice usually appears after four or five days, when physiologic jaundice is receding. If bilirubin levels do not rise too high, then nothing is done and it will resolve itself. Breastfeeding is not interrupted. By the way, there is great debate as to when these levels require treatment and when or if breastfeeding should be interrupted and/or phototherapy begun.

If the bilirubin levels continue to climb beyond 16 mg/dl, your doctor may suggest that you temporarily interrupt breastfeeding for twenty-four to forty-eight hours. Ask if you can alternate breastfeeding and formula every other feeding for a day or so to see if that helps. Sometimes pumped milk that has been heated can be used, too—check on this. If these techniques do not help, then pump your milk every two to three hours and freeze it for later use. This keeps up an adequate milk supply and is only temporary.

If phototherapy is required, ask if this can be done in your home. There are many areas in the country that offer home phototherapy services conducted by a registered nurse in conjunction with your pediatrician.

If your baby is about three to five days old and you are told that he has breast milk jaundice, what this may really be is what we like to call "lack of breastfeeding" jaundice! This means that he is not receiving enough calories and fluid and needs to be nursed more often. Nurse this baby every one to two hours during the day for ten to fifteen minutes per side, if possible. Arbitrary time restrictions on breastfeeding often contribute to the appearance of this condition. If baby won't nurse, pump your milk and feed it to him with a dropper or syringe.

A less common cause of jaundice in the newborn is **ABO incompatibility**. This can occur when the mother has type O blood and the baby has type A, B, or AB blood. It is a situation that sometimes arises during pregnancy if maternal antibodies to these blood types cross the placenta and break down some red blood cells in the baby. This causes a rapid rise in bilirubin levels of the baby soon after birth (the first or second day). Depending on the levels and the rate of rise of bilirubin, the baby may be treated with phototherapy, or in extreme situations, be given a blood transfusion.

Vernix and Lanugo

You may notice a cheese-like substance on your baby's skin. This is called **vernix**. It is a fatty substance secreted by the sebaceous (oil) glands that protects the skin while baby floats in amniotic fluid. Some babies produce a lot of this, others very little.

Vernix generally collects in heavier amounts in the creases and folds of the skin. The body will absorb some of this, some will be wiped or washed off during baths, and the rest can be rubbed into the skin, as it is like a super skin lotion.

You may also have noticed some fine hair across the shoulders, down the spine, or on the upper forehead. This is called **lanugo**, and will rub off in the first week or two. Premature babies generally have more of this fine fuzz.

Your baby may also have dry skin, especially around the wrists and ankles. This is normal and will peel away without anyone's help!

Splotches, Patches, and Spots

New babies can get many types of spots. Thirty to seventy percent of full-term newborn babies can exhibit newborn rash (*erythemia neonatorum toxicum*). This can appear at twenty-four to forty-eight hours of age and disappear in one or two weeks. The spots are red with yellow centers. They form because the baby's skin and pores do not yet work efficiently. These types of spots are not infected and need no treatment, even though they may appear suddenly over the trunk and diaper area.

Mongolian spots are areas of bluish-black pigmentation seen on the lower back and buttocks. They are common in black, oriental, and dark-skinned babies. These spots are temporary accumulations of pigment under the skin and usually fade during the first to second year of life. They have nothing to do with blood disorders, bruises, or Down Syndrome. **Birthmarks** may also concern some parents. If your baby has a birthmark or two, do not feel that it was because of something you have done. Your baby is not "marked" because you had bad thoughts during your pregnancy or went to horror movies or read trashy books! There are many kinds of birthmarks, and only your physician can tell (usually) if they will fade, go away, or remain permanently. Sometimes red marks on the skin are from pressure during the birth and will fade in a few days. Two of the more common birthmarks are called "stork bites" and "strawberry marks."

Stork bites (*Telangiectatic nevi*) are small clusters of pink or red spots found on the nape of the neck, eyelids, and above the bridge of the nose. These are localized areas of capillary dilatation and usually fade by the second birthday. They tend to turn bright réd when baby is angry or crying.

Strawberry marks (*Nevus vascularus*) are newly formed enlarged capillaries that are raised, rough, and dark red, and are usually found in the head region. They grow in size, become fixed by eight months or so, and then begin to regress. They are usually gone by seven years of age. These should be protected from injury, but require no special treatment. Your baby's pediatrician will be able to provide more detailed explanations about these and other less common birth marks.

Maybe your baby does not have any spots. Don't think you're out of the woods yet! Picture this next scene: You think your baby has the most beautiful, clear skin in the world. The baby photographer is coming tomorrow for your free five-by-seven print. Daddy puts baby to bed. Mommy picks up baby for 2 a.m. feeding, and notes in horror that baby's face now looks like a "before" advertisement for an acne treatment product! Baby has pimples all over her face!

Now what happened? Daddy wonders if he did it...when Mom wasn't looking he secretly washed baby's face with the damp dishrag from the sink. Mommy thinks she did it...Baby spit up and she didn't race there fast enough. But it isn't anyone's fault, so don't blame yourselves! Even though you think you can control every aspect of your baby's life, you can't.

What your baby has is a skin rash called **infantile acne**. This condition is caused by an increased level of hormones—like pre-adolescent acne! Please do not call the dermatologist (skin doctor). All babies get this. It will clear up on its own at about twelve weeks of age. There is no treatment for this skin condition.

Grandparents may make a few comments about this. They have forgotten what you looked like at that age. Drag out your own baby pictures and show them your infant acne!

NECK

Please direct your attention to locating your baby's neck. It may be hard to find, but it should be between the chin and the chest. (Most babies look like Cabbage Patch dolls!)

The neck is a prime area for lint collection. We are telling you about this to avoid the embarrassment you feel when the pediatrician or nurse lifts up the chin at the first well-baby checkup and remarks, "Oh, are you saving this lint for something?" You may sink to the floor in embarrassment!

This area is a perfect place for bacteria to thrive. Lift up the chin and wash this area every day, as it is a common place for baby to sweat. Dry it well.

Now, you may think that you have to use lotions, potions, powders, or cornstarch, right? Wrong! This is your choice, but it is not a necessity. And remember, if you want to use powder, do not shake it on baby. The powder can be inhaled by baby and irritate her respiratory system. Powder should be put into your hand first and then applied. If you use cornstarch, be sure that the skin is dry before applying it under the neck—you do not want to glue the chin to the chest! Do babies really need this stuff?

Baby's Layette

Your newborn infant will spend her first several weeks wearing gowns that have drawstrings at the bottom or one-piece suits with feet called "stretchies." There are also stretchies without legs or feet, called "creepers," and kimonos, which are gowns without drawstrings. These outfits are cozy for babies. We recommend that you buy clothing that is too large and let baby grow into it. Otherwise, you will have to buy new clothes for baby every few weeks.

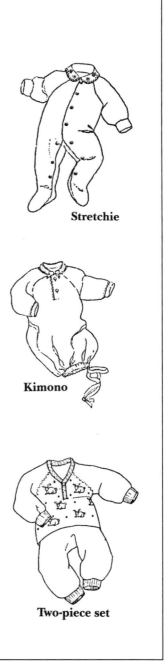

Stretchie

Kimono

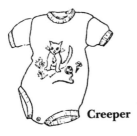

Creeper

Two-piece sets are cute, but the shirts tend to "ride up" on baby's stomach, and you'll want to keep pulling them down.

Infants do not need shoes, especially in the first month. Baby can wear socks or soft knit booties.

Two-piece set

A bonnet will be necessary to keep baby's head warm.

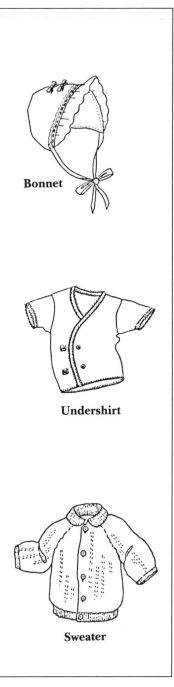

Bonnet

If baby will be wearing cloth diapers, she will need several pairs of plastic waterproof pants to wear over the diapers.

If you will be using cloth diapers and washing them yourself, you will need to buy about four dozen. These four dozen diapers will need to be laundered about twice a week, because baby uses about ninety to one hundred diapers a week.

Undershirts that snap on the side are better than those that have to be pulled over baby's head.

Undershirt

If your baby is born in the winter, she will need a snowsuit. These are one-piece units that zip from the leg to the neck, and they have hoods.

Cotton is the best fabric for baby to wear. It is soft, natural, absorbent, and comfortable. Cotton "breathes," keeping baby cool. Synthetic fabrics trap heat and moisture, and don't launder as well as cotton.

Sweater

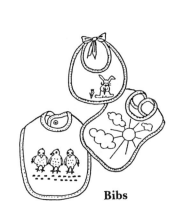

Bibs

A newborn baby who is breastfed will not really need a bib. A bottle-fed baby may wear one, but this is not necessary, either. At this young age, the only thing a bib is used for is to catch spit-up milk—but that usually ends up on *your* clothing as much as baby's! A soft cotton diaper can be placed on your shoulder when you burp baby to catch this spit-up milk. Of course, when baby gets older and starts eating solid foods, bibs are quite necessary.

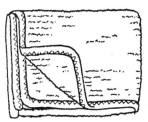

Receiving Blanket

You will definitely need several receiving blankets to wrap baby in, and you will need larger baby blankets, too.

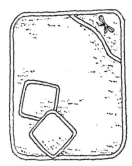

Hooded Bathtowel

A hooded bathtowel is nice to have because you can wrap baby in it immediately after her bath. It will keep her warm, and you can dry her at the same time.

NIPPLES

Nipples are next on our trip down your baby's anatomy. Are they a bit swollen, or do they have a milkish discharge? No, Dad—your son is not lactating! Swollen nipples can be seen in babies of both sexes in the first few days after birth. This condition can last up to two weeks. It is caused by maternal hormones that were intended for Mom but were also received by baby. Some babies have a milky discharge that is called witch's milk.

The nipples should be left alone. Do not attempt to squeeze milk out, thinking that this will make them smaller, as it may cause an infection. The swelling will go away all by itself as baby's body rids itself of these hormones.

UMBILICAL CORD

Now we have arrived at that shriveled cord hanging from your baby's belly. Most parents hope that this will fall off before they leave the hospital. No such luck!

Initially, the cord is white with two umbilical arteries and one umbilical vein that can be easily seen. The cord begins to dry within one to two hours after delivery and is shriveled and blackened by the second or third day. It will fall off within a week or two weeks.

After the cord is clamped at birth, what do we do with it? The clamp will stay on until you leave the hospital, or will be taken off in a couple of days if your stay is longer. When you diaper baby, you should fold the diaper below the navel to help keep it dry. At diaper changes you will usually apply alcohol to the cord stump to encourage it to dry. To clean the cord, just saturate a cotton ball with 10 percent isopropyl or rubbing alcohol and drop two or three drops on the cord. Your baby may cry, not because it burns or stings, but because it is freezing cold. You can also use a cotton swab dipped in alcohol for cord care.

When the cord does fall off, continue to apply alcohol for two to three days to keep the stump dry and the area clean. A small amount of bleeding from the cord stump may be normal. However, if it continues, or if you notice a foul smell from the cord, call your pediatrician. It may need a cauterization (sealing of the capillaries), as a small capillary may not have closed, or it could be infected. Always check with your doctor or nurse practitioner.

GENITALS

When your baby girl or boy is a newborn, you may be quite surprised at how big the genitals seem in proportion to the rest of the body. During the first few days after birth, the scrotum and vulva may be even larger because of maternal hormones that have crossed the placenta and are now causing some swelling. They may also be swollen due to pressures during the birth itself, and may appear red and inflamed. Often these parts may stick out quite a bit. This is normal. The swelling will go down and your child will soon grow into those generous organs!

Little Girls

How do you clean the genital area? All girls (and women too!) should be cleansed from the front to the back. This is to avoid urinary tract and/or vaginal infections from bacteria that normally reside in the stool. If wiped forward, these bacteria can cause an infection. As you wipe gently from front to back, separate the labia and with one damp cotton ball wipe down the right side. With another damp cotton ball wipe down the left side. Use another cotton ball for the rectal area.

Does your daughter have a clear or whitish discharge from her vagina? This is normal and is called "withdrawal bleeding" or **pseudomenstruation**. It may be pink and tinged with blood. It is due to the withdrawal of maternal hormones. Warm water will remove it and keep the area clean.

Little Boys

All boys are born uncircumcised. The decision to circumcise or not is a personal one based on your cultural, religious, and personal beliefs. The American Academy of Pediatrics does not recommend routine circumcision. It is not necessary for your son to match his father or the other boys in the locker room. He will grow up to accept his penis no matter what condition it is in. We hope you feel good about whatever decision you make, because if you don't like the way his penis looks, don't you think he'll get the message?

If you do have your son circumcised, the head of the penis will look red and sore. After the foreskin has been removed, the penis will have gauze and petroleum jelly around it immediately after the procedure. This will fall off in about twenty-four hours. Then, at each diaper change for about five to seven days, apply a small bit of petroleum jelly around the area where the foreskin was removed. The area will heal in about seven to ten days.

If you have chosen not to circumcise, there is no special care for the penis. The penis and foreskin adhere at birth and separate gradually over the first few years of life. You can't retract the foreskin at this age because it is not supposed to be retracted until about three years of age. Don't worry about washing under the foreskin at this age. It is not meant to be cleaned and fussed with from the outside in babyhood. You usually teach your child genital hygiene and toilet education when he is about three years old, anyway. Amazing how nature can put it all together if we just work with it!

Cleaning the genital area is done with a washcloth at diaper changes and bath time. When you clean your son's genital area, be sure to clean under the scrotum, as poop can hide there too!

You also need to know that your son will probably hang on to his penis until he is four or five years old, and he won't go blind! All babies and small children self-stimulate, and it is not harmful. They should feel good about their bodies. If you should find that by about two or three years of age he or she is masturbating a lot, perhaps she is bored. Please buy the child a Big Wheel and get him out for some exercise!

Let's talk about childhood masturbation for a minute. You don't have to worry about this in the first month, but wait until you see your son or daughter masturbating on the potty chair or sitting in front of the T.V. watching Sesame Street! Talk about confronting your great sense of sexual awareness and permissiveness! It always amazes us that people talk about how open they are when it comes to sexual matters, but can't handle masturbation in their children. "What should we do?" "Will he go blind?" "What did we do wrong?" Think about your own morals and relax. You want your child to feel good about his body. In many ways we really grow up through our children. You think that all your defenses are mature and healthy—well, you have met your match! Your child will confront every part of your personality and development. The pure, naive honesty of children makes you rethink and reformulate your responses.

THE EXTREMITIES—FEET AND HANDS

As a newborn, your baby's hands and feet may remain a little blue or mottled in coloring for a few days until the capillaries (small blood vessels) open fully. This is normal. But what about those fingernails? They grow quickly and may already extend beyond the ends of the fingers.

Your baby's nails will be very soft for the first few days, because he lived in an aquatic environment for nine months. It will take about seven to ten days for his nails to harden.

The nails will not be cut while the baby is in the hospital. This is because they are so soft and adhere tightly to the underlying skin, so if you cut them there is a good chance that you will cut the skin and open up an area to infection. Usually the baby is kept in a long-sleeved t-shirt that has little cuffs at the ends of the sleeves. These cuffs are pulled over the baby's hands to prevent him from scratching his face. Please don't leave baby's hands covered for too long. Those fingers touching the face are an important part of baby's development.

After you get home there are several ways that mothers can handle these nails.

- Bite them off! Your lips are more sensitive than your fingers or scissors and can more easily tell where the nail ends and the finger begins.
- Use an emery board to gently file the ragged edges.
- Gently peel them away as they separate from the underlying skin.
- Put baby on her tummy. She will scratch the sheets, causing the nails to fold over so they are easier to peel off.

In seven to ten days, when the nails are harder, you can cut them with small, blunt-tipped scissors. The scissor tips must be rounded to prevent cutting the skin. Do not use nail clippers, as you cannot judge nail from skin with these. It is easier at first to clip nails with another adult holding the baby's hand or foot still. An even better idea is to clip the nails while the baby is in a deep sleep. Babies hate getting their nails cut.

So far, we have been looking at the outside of baby and some of what it takes to care for the exterior. You will find yourself constantly aware of many of the exterior changes that occur as your baby grows. The only thing that is constant about children is that they are always changing. You may wonder how you're going to remember all of this or have time to figure things out. Much of your time, though, will be directed toward taking care of the "interior" of baby—that is, feeding him! This is covered in the next chapter of Parenthood 101.

Chapter Two
Feeding Your Baby

After you have a baby, your two most common activities will be changing diapers and feeding the baby. You may choose to breastfeed, bottle feed, or use a combination of both.

Most parents decide how they will feed their baby during the middle to late part of the pregnancy. Some are undecided right to the end! In this section we will look at feeding choices and explore techniques to help make feedings enjoyable for all of you.

You will find that how and what you feed your baby will generate more comments than almost anything else (except crying!). Parents choose to breast- or bottle feed for many reasons. What we want to do is give you a look at each feeding method and how combination feeding works, so that you can either make your decision or feel more comfortable with the decision you have already made.

The information in this section is based on the most current research available, with a bias toward breastfeeding. We give you this information after many years of working with new families and thousands of hours in our own clinical practices. We do not intend to make this a "fight" between breastfeeding and bottle feeding. It is not a fight, but it is often a decision based on opinion.

COMMON MISCONCEPTIONS ABOUT BREASTFEEDING

- **Breastfeeding is animal-like**. How else are mammals supposed to feed their young?

- **Why bother? It's easier to give a bottle.** Maybe, maybe not.
- **Breastfeeding is messy!** Try cleaning up a bottle or a can of spilled formula, and scrubbing ten nipples, bottles, rings, and caps every day.
- **Breastfeeding is disgusting—any fluid that comes out of the body is dirty.** Breastmilk is the most nutritious food you can give your baby.
- **You will expose your breasts and it will be embarrassing.** For whom? Have you been to the beach lately?
- **You'll be tied down.** Where are you going? You will always be tied down when you have children, no matter how you feed them.
- **You can't go back to work if you breastfeed.** The majority of women in the world work and nurse.
- **"I didn't or couldn't do it, so why should you?"** Many women who have had unpleasant or discouraging experiences with breastfeeding say this as they try to convince themselves that what they did was right. They feel uncomfortable with the idea that you might succeed where they failed. Usually they just didn't have the right kind of help. When these people talk to you about breastfeeding they may be full of anger and guilt rather than support. Sympathize with them, but realize that your experience will bear no relationship to theirs.

MYTHS AND OLD WIVES' TALES

My breasts are too small, too large, or not the same size.

The size of your breasts does not determine their functional capacity. Size is related to fat content, not the number of milk-making glands. It doesn't matter what size your breasts are. As long as they undergo the changes caused by pregnancy, they will produce plenty of milk.

My nipples are too small or too large, the areola is too large—how will all this fit into baby's mouth?

The size of the nipples and areola has nothing to do with success at breastfeeding. It is not necessary, nor is it possible, to put the entire areola into the baby's mouth. Only the nipple and one-half inch or so of the areola goes into baby's mouth. But flat or inverted nipples are a factor that can possibly interfere with smooth breastfeeding.

My breasts will sag and hang down to my knees if I breastfeed.

The hormonally caused changes of *pregnancy*, not nursing, determine what the breasts will look like after weaning. Heredity, nutrition, and exercise also contribute to this. The fat in the breasts is what gives them their size and shape. The fat is replaced by glandular tissue during pregnancy. Once the milk is gone from the breasts, the fat does not return to resculpt the breasts.

I'll lose my figure or get it back faster if I do/do not breastfeed.

Breastfeeding will use two to three hundred calories per day from fat stores laid down during pregnancy. With sensible nutrition and exercise you will regain your figure as well as anyone else. This is highly individual. You may not lose the last couple of pounds until you wean the baby, as this is water that the body wants to retain.

I'm too nervous, high strung, and tense, so I won't make enough milk.

This has nothing to do with milk production. Sometimes real tension or anxiety will slow down the delivery of milk. Usually, finding and alleviating the cause of the tension, as well as the use of relaxation techniques, plus confidence, helps with the situation.

The father will be left out and won't be able to parent the baby.

There is more to parenting than putting food in a child's mouth. The love a father has for his child can be communicated in many ways, such as changing, dressing, holding, rocking, walking, bathing, and talking. Show baby your hobbies, work on the car engine, sit him in front of your computer terminal, read him the newspaper—babies don't care! Lie down for a nap with baby on your chest. This is better than a $2,000 brass crib! Play with your baby—they thrive on this!

MISINFORMATION

Misinformation about how to breastfeed a baby abounds among your friends, relatives, and even with health care professionals. Use the breastfeeding information here and refer to the breast-feeding resources listed at the end of this book for a good start. Beware of people who tell you that there is only one way to do things. Avoid strict schedules and rules that do not allow flexibility for the individual variations found in all babies.

THE BUTTINSKIS

The Buttinskis are a family who know all, and are not shy about telling you exactly what you should and should not do. They come out of the woodwork as soon as you walk by with a pregnant abdomen or a new baby. They are often strangers, or just acquaintances who feel compelled to tell you how to do things—especially how to feed a baby. Sometimes they are family members who have you under a microscope. Be polite, tell them you'll consider what they say, thank them for their interest, then do what you want! You are the parents!

WHY BREASTFEED?

There are many things that are good about breastfeeding, both for you and for the baby. Let's look at these briefly. They make good ammunition for use with the Buttinskis. And it never hurts to tell them that you are doing what you are doing because you just plain want to!

The nutritional components that occur in **colostrum** (the first milk from the breast) and breast milk are the right kind and amount, and occur at the right time, in keeping with the needs and stores of a new baby. Breast milk is easier to digest, does not put a heavy load on baby's excretory system, and changes composition to meet baby's varying needs. Colostrum and mother's milk contain special anti-infective properties that protect baby against many diseases and infections.

Colostrum has a laxative effect on baby, which hastens the elimination of **meconium** (the black tar-like first bowel movement). Meconium is laden with bilirubin, which contributes to newborn jaundice. Frequent colostrum feedings decrease the incidence and severity of newborn or physiologic jaundice.

Breast milk is also anti-allergenic and this is important. A nursing baby will not be allergic to his own mother's milk. A family with a positive history of allergies needs to seriously consider breastfeeding their baby. In addition, breast milk is clean, portable, and inexpensive, and never needs to be mixed, fixed, heated, or cooled.

There are no disadvantages to a baby in feeding him breast milk. Sometimes the mother will anticipate inconveniences and see these as disadvantages. The inconveniences are that there may be minor physical discomfort, it takes some time to learn the art and skill of breastfeeding, and you need to be around for feedings during the early learning period. These are temporary concerns and can be handled with patience, time, correct information, and support.

WHY BOTTLEFEED?

Parents often choose formula feeding because of misinformation, incorrect management of breastfeeding, outside commitments, or simply because they want to bottle feed. What is important is that your choice be an informed one.

Breastfed babies can be given bottles when it is not convenient for Mom to stay home and nurse. Bottles of expressed breast milk or formula can be kept on hand so that Mom can get out of the house or return to work without stopping the breastfeeding process. Formula can be expensive, needs refrigeration, and may not agree with baby. Breast milk needs to be refrigerated, but is free, and always agrees with baby. All bottle feeding equipment must be washed and/or sterilized, which means more time in the kitchen for you.

In the end, you must do what you feel is right for you. If you are undecided, try breastfeeding. You can always switch to a bottle if it is not for you. It's a little more difficult (but possible) to go from bottlefeeding to breastfeeding.

BEGINNING TO BREASTFEED

You may be surprised the first time you put your baby to your breast. Your baby may prefer to just lick or nuzzle the nipple rather than actually feed. You may feel that you need eight hands to position him comfortably! Or, your baby may latch right on and enjoy his first meal very soon after birth. Both of these situations are normal.

Breastfeeding is an art and a skill that is learned by both you and your baby. As with any new skill, the more you practice, the better you will become. And you will have lots of time to practice! The following information will help you get off to a good start by answering some of your questions, explaining how breastfeeding works, and teaching you some basic breastfeeding techniques.

Understanding Lactation (Breastfeeding)

Knowing a little about lactation will help you understand how to work with your body and why the guidelines here will encourage a successful breastfeeding experience.

The Equipment

The breasts are specialized organs that undergo changes during pregnancy in preparation for breastfeeding. They increase in size as the milk-making and delivering apparatus develop.

Milk is made in special sacs called **alveoli**. The alveoli are surrounded by special little cells that push the milk out and down the ducts to the nipple when the baby nurses. The milk collects in widened milk sinuses behind the nipple and beneath the **areola** (the large, dark circle of tissue surrounding the nipple). The baby removes the milk from these sinuses or reservoirs by the special way he sucks at breast.

The Process

Once the **placenta** (afterbirth) has been delivered, a hormonal change occurs in your body that allows your breasts to begin producing milk. There are two parts to lactation: the making of milk and the giving of milk. The size of your breasts is not related to either of these.

Your breasts make milk by following the law of supply and demand—the more milk removed, the more milk you make. When your baby sucks on the nipple and areola, a message is sent to your brain that stimulates the release of a hormone called **oxytocin**. Oxytocin causes the little cells around the alveoli to contract and push the milk out and down to the milk sinuses behind the areola. This is called the **letdown reflex** or **milk ejection reflex**. The baby's nursing action also causes another hormone called **prolactin** to be released. Prolactin is the hormone that tells the breasts to make more milk.

The First Feedings

Most babies are awake and alert for about an hour or two following their birth. This is an ideal time for you and your baby to start learning about nursing.

The first food your baby receives from the breast is called colostrum. It is a yellowish fluid that contains anti-infective factors which help protect your baby from disease. Colostrum is special food for a new baby's first few days of life as the protein, sugar, and fat occur in forms and quantities that are very easy to digest. Colostrum will gradually change over a few days to milk.

Breast milk seen at the beginning of a feeding generally looks thin and watery. This is called **foremilk** and accumulates in the milk sinuses between feedings. After the milk ejection reflex (letdown) has occurred during a feeding, the milk will look thicker and creamier. This is the **hindmilk**, which contains a higher amount of fat.

How Frequently Should Baby Be Fed?

You will feed your baby as soon after birth as possible, and about every two or three hours thereafter during the day. The baby will wake once or more during the night in the early weeks. The range of feedings is about eight to twelve times in twenty-four hours. Some mothers feed their babies very frequently during the day to decrease the number of night feedings. Do not let the baby sleep longer than about four hours between feedings during the day or about six hours at night during the early weeks. It is important to feed your baby this frequently as breast milk is rapidly digested and used by the baby. The components of human milk occur in such a way that frequent feedings are required to maintain the health and growth of a rapidly developing infant. Your baby will need to be fed every two or three hours in the early weeks, until he is able to stretch out feedings.

As baby gets older, these nursing patterns change. After the first six weeks or so, your baby may start to go longer between some of the feedings and sleep a little longer at night. *This is different for all babies!*

Many mothers feed their babies "on demand." This is fine, as long as the baby "demands" to be fed eight to twelve times in twenty-four hours. Some babies do not indicate hunger very noisily or just prefer to sleep. These quieter babies must be awakened and fed just as much as their noisier neighbors!

There are no rules here. Each baby is unique. Use your common sense—if the baby is hungry, feed him. If you try to stretch out feedings beyond what the baby can tolerate, then baby ends up doing a lot of crying and may not gain weight, and you end up frustrated and crying, too.

Normal, healthy, full-term babies do not need supplementary bottles of formula or sugar water. These are unnecessary and can confuse your baby's feeding patterns during the learning period. Breastfed babies do not need to be given water at all. Only under special circumstances are additional fluids necessary. These circumstances would be when a baby has low blood sugar (infant of a diabetic mother), low birth weight, or has experienced unusual stress at delivery. Occasionally your pediatrician will recommend supplementary water for a bottle-fed baby, especially if the baby is constipated. Bottles of water or formula can do the following.

- Suppress baby's appetite, causing baby to nurse less frequently.
- Change the way baby's mouth is positioned at breast.
- Condition baby to nurse only on a long solid nipple.
- Cause tongue thrust, which pushes the nipple and areola out of baby's mouth.
- Decrease baby's willingness to nurse long enough to cause

the milk ejection (letdown) reflex, since formula and water flow rapidly and immediately from the large hole in a bottle nipple.

- Risk intolerance or allergies to formula in susceptible babies.
- Give you the message that you or the breastfeeding process is not adequate for your baby.

How Long Should Feedings Last?

Again, there are no rules here. Usually it is the baby who determines how long he will nurse, as he knows when he is full! However, in the early weeks, some babies are not very efficient at nursing, or fall asleep at the breast. This means that it may take them longer than you think to withdraw enough milk for their needs.

Many mothers are told to limit the number of minutes that they nurse in order to prevent sore nipples. Sore nipples have five main causes, none of which is related to how long a baby nurses. These are discussed on page 40.

As a general guide, nurse seven to ten minutes on each side at each feeding right from the start. Some babies will nurse longer, some shorter. This is highly individual. If baby is nursing in the correct position, you may notice a little tenderness when he first latches on, but this quickly disappears during the feeding. There is no need to limit sucking time if baby is positioned correctly and you are comfortable. By the time your milk comes in (twelve to forty-eight hours after delivery), your baby will probably have decided how long he needs to nurse, whether it be ten minutes per side or twenty minutes per side. They are all different!

You will offer both breasts at each feeding and start on the side where the previous feeding ended. When you remove baby from the breast, be sure that you break the suction by inserting your little finger into the side of the baby's mouth to prevent undue stress on the nipple.

Spitting Up and Burping

Most babies spit up. You may notice a spurt of milk when baby burps or see milk trickling down baby's chin after or between feedings. This occurs when the lower esophageal or cardiac sphincter (the last five centimeters of the esophagus before the stomach) remains relaxed rather than constricted and allows milk to reflux or back up into the esophagus. As the baby's digestive system matures, he will outgrow this. The following are suggestions for dealing with this situation.

- Avoid overfeeding baby.
- Time feedings so baby is not over-hungry. When he is over-hungry, he gulps his feedings, and swallows air.
- Use short, frequent feedings of smaller amounts of milk.
- Burp baby before a feeding, especially if he has been crying.
- Burp baby frequently during a feeding as well as after feedings.
- Place baby at a 35–45° angle in a baby seat for thirty minutes following feedings.
- Place baby on his right side to sleep.

Some babies spit up frequently, even several times during or after a feeding. This usually looks like an enormous amount of milk but is more like a tablespoon of fluid. If baby spits up more than you are comfortable with, or if there is a great deal of force behind the milk so that it is ejected a couple of feet, contact your pediatric nurse practitioner or pediatrician to have this checked.

Breastfed babies should be burped between breasts and after each feeding. Bottlefed babies should be burped about halfway through the feeding and after the feeding. As mentioned above, babies who are irritable while being fed should be burped several times during and after the feeding. (You may wish to place a cotton diaper on your shoulder, if that is how you are burping baby, to catch spit-up milk.) See Figure 2.1 for burping positions.

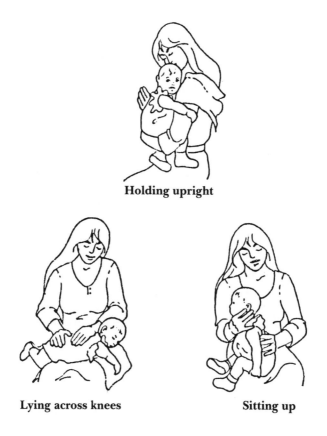

Holding upright

Lying across knees   **Sitting up**

Figure 2.1.   Positions to Use When Burping Your Baby

Positioning Yourself and Your Baby

You can comfortably nurse in many positions, including the following.

1.   Position yourself comfortably before you nurse the baby. In the hospital, elevate the back of the bed, and put a pillow behind your head and back and another pillow on your lap. Raise your knees with a pillow under them, or raise your hospital bed so that your knees are elevated. This allows you to bring the baby closer to the breast without leaning

forward. Leaning down to nurse a baby can lead to back strain and cracked nipples.

Place the baby on his side on top of the pillow in your lap with his legs wrapped around your waist. Arrange your arm so that the shoulder and elbow are in a straight line with the bent elbow directly in front of the nipple cradling the baby's head. You and the baby will be chest to chest and his head will not have to turn sideways to reach the nipple. Figure 2.2 illustrates this position.

2. You can nurse while lying on your side by placing baby on his side with his whole body facing you. His mouth will be level with the nipple. Do not allow him to pull down on the nipple to nurse. See Figure 2.3.

3. A third position that is often used is called the football hold. Place a pillow at your side and sit the baby facing the breast with his mouth at the level of the nipple. This may be an easier position for you to learn how to breastfeed as it gives you better control of baby's head. It is also easier to see what you are doing. See Figure 2.4 for an example of the football hold.

Putting Baby to Breast

After you have found a comfortable position, follow these steps to put baby to breast.

1. Place four fingers of your free hand under your breast to support its weight, and place your thumb lightly just above and beyond the edge of the areola.

2. Stimulate the baby's rooting reflex by touching your nipple to the baby's lower lip. (See Figure 1.2.) As baby opens his mouth, bring him up closer (do not lean down) and lift the breast up a little to guide the nipple in. It will take a few tries to coordinate all this! If baby does not open his mouth wide enough or long enough, use the index finger of the hand supporting your breast to pull down on baby's lower lip or chin.

3. Once your baby has the nipple and about one-half inch of the areola in his mouth, you can tip the nipple up toward the roof of his mouth if he does not suck. It is not necessary,

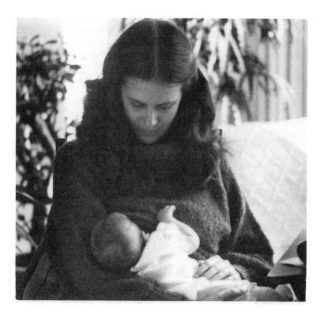

Figure 2.2. Breastfeeding in the Sitting Position

nor is it possible, to stuff the entire areola into a baby's mouth! The gums just need to be positioned over the milk sinuses.

4. Place the index finger of the hand holding the breast under baby's chin. This supports his chin and jaw to help him keep hold of the nipple. Keep your other fingers under your breast to support its weight so that the heavy tissue does not cause baby to keep losing the nipple.

5. If baby loses the nipple or if nursing is painful, remove baby and reposition him.

6. Burp baby between sides and after feedings. He may or may not have a burp, but always try! Sitting him up, burping him, or switching sides will help wake him and renew his interest in nursing if he is sleepy. Some mothers switch sides frequently during a feeding if baby is falling asleep on the first breast and not taking the second.

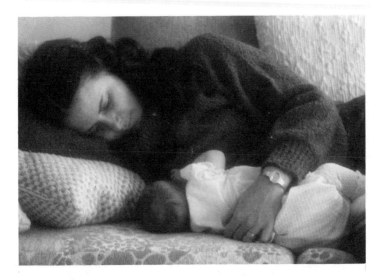

Figure 2.3.   Breastfeeding While Lying Down

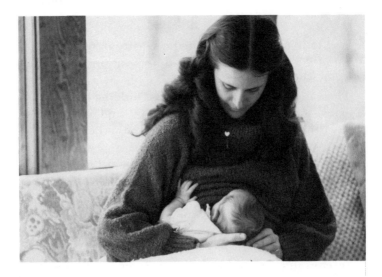

Figure 2.4.   Breastfeeding Using the Football Hold

Nipple Care

Air-dry your nipples for ten minutes or so after each feeding before you close the bra flaps. Do not use soap, alcohol (or products that contain alcohol), petroleum-based products, or any other goops on your nipples. Lanolin and vitamin E oil are not necessary either, and do not prevent or cure sore nipples. Improper positioning is usually the cause of real soreness. If you are leaking milk, do not wear nursing pads with plastic liners or allow the nipples to sit for long periods of time in wet pads. This breaks down nipple tissue and can cause soreness. Do not wear plastic milk cups for leaking, as these just encourage more milk to leak and can cause your nipples to become sore from the moisture buildup.

How Will I Know if Baby is Getting Enough Milk?

Most new mothers wonder if their baby is receiving enough milk. Relatives and friends often ask this question whenever the baby cries! Several indications of a well-fed baby are listed below.

- Eight or more wet diapers in twenty-four hours after the first week (with no supplemental water being given).
- Clear, pale urine (not dark yellow and concentrated).
- Eight to twelve feedings in twenty-four hours.
- One or more bowel movements per day. (Some babies save up for a couple of days and have enormous bowel movements a little less frequently.)
- You see milk and *hear baby swallowing* during feedings.
- A steady weight gain of between four and eight ounces per week.

Weight gain is a highly individual process, and many breastfed babies take two or three weeks to regain their birth weight. The scale sometimes becomes the indicator of a mother's success at nurturing her child. Some babies, however, channel their calories into growth in length at first, and later catch up on weight gain. Your baby's growth is measured not only in weight, but also in length and head circumference. You have not "failed" as a mother if your baby does not gain weight rapidly. If you are nursing frequently for a sufficient length of time, if baby is not just gumming or dozing at the breast, and if you are well-nourished and rested, then your baby is probably following an inherited pattern of weight gain. If there is any question regarding adequate weight gain, consult your pediatrician or nurse practitioner to make sure that baby is not ill. A professional lactation consultant can help discover and correct faulty nursing patterns or ineffective breastfeeding techniques.

Some mothers think that they are losing their milk in the early weeks when their breasts become smaller and softer. The normal swelling that accompanies the beginning of milk production (engorgement) will disappear, but not the milk! This reduction in the swelling of the breasts often occurs at a time when the baby seems to want to nurse more frequently (when he is about seven to fourteen days old). This could lead one to suspect that there is not enough milk. What is usually happening is that the baby is experiencing a growth spurt. These occur periodically as the need for milk increases to support the baby's high rate of growth. Growth spurts can occur at any time, but are typically seen around ten days following the birth, at four to six weeks of age, around three months, and at six months. At these times, the baby seems as if he is never filled up. By nursing frequently, your baby is stimulating the production of the additional milk that he needs to continue growing.

COMMON PROBLEMS IN THE FIRST FEW WEEKS OF BREASTFEEDING

Most mothers find that nursing their baby is an enjoyable and satisfying experience. Once the milk supply is well established and the nursing relationship is going well, most mothers will not experience problems with the actual mechanisms of lactation (breastfeeding). There are, however, some situations that may arise early in the nursing experience that new mothers should be aware of. Not every mother will experience any or all of these problems, but it is important to be aware that they exist and to know both how to avoid them and how to handle them if they occur. This awareness will help you gain confidence in yourself in the early weeks of breastfeeding.

It is important to remember that these situations are usually minor and temporary. They can often be avoided by proper prevention techniques, or successfully handled by immediate treatment. The following is a discussion of some of the more common obstacles that may be encountered during the "learning" period of the early weeks. Suggestions are offered for preventing and handling these situations to help make your nursing experience stress-free and satisfying.

Engorgement

Engorgement (the swelling of the breasts) is a normal and temporary condition that usually occurs between two to five days following the birth of your baby. All newly delivered women become engorged. If this is not your first baby, this may occur in twelve to twenty-four hours. It is caused by a combination of factors that are preparing your breasts to begin making milk. These factors include an increase in the blood supply to the breasts, an increased amount of fluid in the breast tissues, and a buildup of pressure in the milk ducts as a result of milk being made but not being removed. If this normal engorgement is unrelieved because milk is not being removed, then severe engorgement can occur, and this condition is extremely painful. Let's look at the this condition and how to handle it.

Signs of Normal Engorgement

- The engorged breasts may feel full, heavy, and swollen.
- An engorged breast may be sensitive to the touch.
- The nipple may flatten out and be hard for baby to grasp as the areola fills with milk.
- You may have a low grade fever (99–101°F), feel achey, or have a slight headache.
- The breasts may feel warm and your bra may fit very snugly.

Severe Engorgement

Severely engorged breasts will be very painful all the way into the underarm area. They may feel rock hard, hot to the touch, and the skin may appear very shiny. It may be difficult for you to

find a comfortable position to sit or lie in. Severe, painful engorgement can be prevented.

Preventing Painful Engorgement

- To prevent painful engorgement, nurse your baby soon after
  birth and frequently thereafter. Plan to feed your baby about
  every two to three hours during the day or on demand,
  whichever comes first. Nursing every two or three hours will
  encourage the milk to come in sooner, adequately nourish
  your baby, and prevent the milk from backing up and causing the breasts to become more severely engorged. If your
  breasts become overfull, your baby will have a difficult time
  attaching to the nipple and will probably place his mouth on
  the nipple in a rather awkward position. This incorrect position causes the nipples to become sore. Your breasts can
  become full when the milk comes in, but will not become
  painfully engorged if they are frequently and adequately
  drained. If the baby nurses lazily or sleeps through a feeding, be sure to express the milk from your breast either by
  hand or with a good manual or electric pump.
- Nurse your baby at least once during the night to prevent
  your breasts from becoming overfull. Have him brought to
  you from the nursery when he awakens, even if it is not on
  the hospital's schedule. Request that your baby not be given
  any sugar water or formula between feedings. The sugar
  suppresses baby's appetite and lengthens the interval between feedings (and therefore the draining of the breasts).
  This supplemental feeding of sugar water or formula may
  also cause nipple confusion and discourage baby from nursing at the breast.
- Do not skip or delay feedings. If your baby does not awaken
  about every two to three hours, try to wake and nurse him
  when he moves or makes noises in his sleep, or when you see
  mouthing or sucking movements or rapid eye movements
  under the eyelids. Some babies are very sleepy, but still need
  to be fed. Also, many babies do not cry when they want to be
  fed.
- Do not restrict sucking time to just two to three minutes at
  each breast. Nurse between seven and ten minutes on each

side at each feeding right from the start. Limiting the amount of time that your baby sucks will not necessarily prevent sore nipples. What it can do is lead to breasts that are not adequately drained because the baby did not nurse long enough to activate the letdown (milk-ejection) reflex, which pushes the milk down to the nipple. As the engorged breast continues to fill with milk, the nipple will flatten out and become difficult for the baby to grasp properly. If enough pressure is built up from lack of milk removal it will be harder to remove milk and will ultimately decrease the milk making capacity of your breast.

- Offer both breasts at each feeding. Start the next feeding on the breast you ended with at the last feeding.

Managing Engorgement

- Arrange short, frequent feedings, every one-and-a-half to two hours for about five to seven minutes on each side.
- Although we usually discourage the use of milk cups, with this condition it may help to use them between feedings to relieve pressure by allowing excess milk to drip out. The milk will stop dripping after the pressure is relieved. Empty these cups and wash them frequently. Do not save or give baby this collected milk.
- Apply moist heat to your breasts for ten or fifteen minutes before each feeding. You can stand in a hot shower with your back to the water, allowing it to run over your breasts. Hot, wet washcloths can be used as compresses on the breast. An even more effective technique is to submerge the breasts in a bowl or sink of hot water. Cold packs can be applied following feedings for temporary pain relief, but this does not relieve engorgement.
- Follow the moist heat with breast massage. Massage from the outer parts of the breasts toward the nipple or with small circular motions once or twice around the breasts. Next, hand express or pump out a little milk to soften the areola and make it easier for your baby to grasp. You can also use the hospital's electric breast pump or a good hand pump.
- Do not use nipple shields. These are nipple-shaped rubber or silicone devices that are placed over your nipples. The baby

attaches to these shields during feedings. These will only serve to decrease stimulation to the breasts and can damage nipples, confuse your baby's sucking pattern, and prevent the breast from being adequately drained. This can also lead to a decrease in the milk supply and weight gain in baby.

- Massage the breasts during feedings to encourage milk flow.
- Painful engorgement is best treated by prevention.

Sore Nipples

Many women are concerned that nursing will be painful, and think that if they are blond or have fair skin it will be even worse. This section will look at nipple discomfort and what can be done about it.

First of all, the color of your hair or skin type has nothing to do with nipple soreness. Second, not all women experience nipple pain when they nurse. Many women find that their nipples are somewhat sensitive and tender for the first week or two, especially when the baby first latches on at each feeding. This tenderness generally disappears after about two weeks when the nipples are accustomed to the nursing action. This type of soreness is normal in a culture where the nipples are always covered. It lasts only a short period of time and will not keep you from enjoying a pleasant breastfeeding experience.

Soreness beyond this can be caused by any of the conditions listed below.

- Undiagnosed or uncorrected flat or inverted nipples.
- Severe engorgement. (See pages 38 and 39 for treatment and prevention of this condition.)
- Poor positioning of baby at breast.
- Baby's improper sucking pattern.

Flat or Inverted Nipples

Check for and begin to correct this condition if it exists. Perform the "pinch test" to determine if your nipples protrude far enough to be properly grasped by your baby. The "pinch test" mimics what your nipple will do when your baby nurses. Compress the areola (the brown circle of tissue that surrounds the nipple) between your thumb and forefinger. If the nipple sticks out, even a little way, then this should not pose a problem for the baby. However, if your nipple flattens to the level of the areola or folds into the areolar tissue, then the nipple is flat and will be difficult for the baby to grasp. Your baby may have a hard time removing milk from the breast, and the improper sucking technique on this type of nipple can make it very sore. Be sure to check both nipples.

Management

- Obtain and wear a milk cup or breast shell. This is a device that comes in two parts and is worn under your bra. The flat piece has a hole in the middle through which the nipple will protrude and which is placed directly over the nipple first. After the flat piece is in place, attach the dome cover to it and pull up the bra flap. When this is done, a very gentle pressure is exerted at the base of the nipple, which encourages it to become more protrusive. Wear these cups between feedings, removing them a couple of times during the day to prevent moisture buildup. Remove them at bedtime. Discard any milk that collects in the cups and wash them in hot soapy water, rinse well, and allow them to air dry. If your cups have only one hole in the dome, more can be drilled for better ventilation. Breast shells need to have plenty of holes to allow air to circulate.
- Pull the nipple out and roll it between the fingers before each feeding. This shapes the nipple to better fit in baby's mouth. A little ice applied to the nipple sometimes helps too.
- One of the best techniques to help draw out flat nipples is to use a good manual or electric pump for a few minutes before each feeding. This will draw out the nipple, soften the areola by removing milk, and start the milk flowing as an incentive for baby to continue working to grasp the nipple.

Poor Positioning of Baby at Breast

This is probably the most frequent cause of severely sore or cracked nipples.

Signs

- Pain that lasts throughout the feeding, not just at latch on.
- Cracks or fissures on the top, sides or bottom of the nipple that, if deep enough, may bleed.
- If your baby takes a long time to latch on or pulls or arches off the breast, then you need to adjust your position.
- Your position is improper if you are leaning down over the baby while nursing rather than having your baby high up and on his side level with the breast. The baby should come to the breast—don't lean down to bring the breast to the baby.

Prevention and Management

- Short, frequent feedings, every two or three hours for seven to ten minutes per side or every one or two hours for five minutes per side.
- Place a pillow on your lap with the baby lying on his side (chest to chest) and with his mouth at the level of your nipple. Baby's head will not be turned to the side. His whole body faces your body.
- You can alternate feeding positions by placing a pillow at your side and sitting baby on the pillow, facing your breast with his mouth at the level of the nipple (this is called the football hold; see Figure 2.4).
- Do not lean over or draw away from the baby as he approaches the nipple.
- Do not use creams, ointments, or vitamin E oil on sore or cracked nipples, as this seals out the air and prolongs the healing time. These products do not prevent or cure sore nipples. Just express some breast milk on the nipples and allow this to air dry.
- Support your breast with the opposite hand when you nurse. Place four fingers under your breast and lift gently to help keep the nipple in baby's mouth.

Baby's Improper Sucking Pattern

Some babies develop a pattern of nursing that can be very damaging to the nipples.

Signs

- You feel pain during the feeding, not just at latch on.
- Baby's cheeks draw inward and dimple while nursing.
- Baby's tongue is not on his lower gum but may be pulled back or upward.
- Clicking or smacking sounds are heard as baby nurses.
- Baby bites down as soon as the nipple touches his mouth rather than opening wide and drawing in the nipple and one-half inch or so of the areola.
- The tip of the nipple is white when removed from baby's mouth.
- Slow weight gain and excessive fussiness on the baby's part.
- Baby's mouth does not form a complete seal at the breast (inadequate suction).
- Rapid movements of baby's head back and forth at breast, crying at breast.

Management of Improper Sucking Pattern

- Proper positioning, as described above.
- Open baby's mouth for him by pulling down on his chin or lower lip as he is put to breast.
- Lift up the breast with the three supporting fingers and slip the forefinger under baby's chin to hold it in place.
- Put your finger in baby's mouth to push the tongue down onto the lower gum and calm him before placing him at breast.
- Express some milk onto your nipple or into baby's mouth to encourage him to open wide.

Leaking

The leaking of milk is more of an annoyance than a problem. It is temporary, and is generally the result of milk letting down at inappropriate times. Some mothers will let down or eject milk

General Nipple Care

- No soap, alcohol, or other drying agents should be applied to the nipples.
- No creams, ointments, tea bags, "goops," or vitamin E oil will prevent or cure sore nipples.
- Do not use nipple shields (or bottle nipples) that cover your nipples while baby nurses.
- Break suction properly when removing baby from breast. Insert your little finger between baby's gums to avoid pulling and stress on the nipple.
- Air-dry nipples following each feeding. Make sure the nipples are completely dry before attaching the bra flap. Do not let the nipples sit in wet nursing pads if you are leaking milk.

between feedings or when just hearing a baby cry or thinking of their own infant. It is more common to see this in a mother who is nursing for the first time. This could be because the milk reservoirs behind the areola have not yet stretched to accommodate much storage of milk between feedings. Or perhaps, the closure mechanism around the nipple pores does not work well at first.

Leaking Between Feedings

If your breasts are leaking milk between feedings, you can use breast pads that are either washable cotton or disposable without plastic liners. Some mothers use folded handkerchiefs or cut up cloth diapers to protect their clothing. These should be worn only if necessary and changed very frequently. Nipples that are allowed to sit in wet pads can become very sore.

Do not wear milk cups to catch leaking milk. They put pressure on the areola and cause further leaking. They may also allow moisture to build up and cause the nipples to become sore. The milk that collects in these cups should not be given to the baby because it may contain high amounts of bacteria.

When milk lets down unexpectedly, you can press the heel of your hand firmly against the nipple or cross your arms over your breasts and press back toward your chest to stop the flow of milk.

The leaking will gradually stop by six to eight weeks, and often much sooner.

Leaking During Feedings

While the baby nurses at one breast, milk often leaks from the other. This is a good sign, since it shows that milk is letting down. You can press the heel of your hand against the nipple or use your arm to prevent the milk from leaking out. Some experienced mothers will collect the leaking milk in a bottle or pump it with a battery-operated or electric pump in order to save milk or increase their milk supply.

You can place a diaper under the leaking breast while nursing to avoid getting your clothes wet. You can also tape a nurser bag to the breast to collect the milk.

Blisters

Sometimes nursing mothers notice a blister on the tip of the nipple. It may be filled with clear fluid or blood. Such blisters can result from a vigorously sucking baby or from poor positioning at the breast. They usually disappear by themselves as the skin becomes accustomed to the nursing action. If they break or become painful, try changing the baby's position at breast so that different areas of the nipple and areola are subject to the strongest point of stress. You can also apply a warm, wet washcloth to the blister before nursing. This will help soften it so it will not crack. Be sure to start feedings on the unaffected side. Make sure you are not holding the nipple and areola in a "v" with your fingers, and see that baby takes more of the areola into his mouth.

Plugged Ducts

Plugged or clogged ducts is a condition that many nursing mothers will experience at one time or another. This can occur if milk is not being removed on a frequent and regular basis or if the milk is being obstructed in its flow to the nipple. Plugged ducts can be felt through the skin as small lumps or large areas of hardness. It is important that you remedy this situation quickly, as milk that is left pooled in a clog can sometimes cause a breast infection.

Signs

- You may experience a small area of tenderness on a breast.
- Often you can feel a lump in the sore area. That is the plug.

Prevention

- Frequent, regular nursing or pumping of the breasts is important to keep the milk flowing.
- Do not wear bras with underwire supports as these may restrict the flow of milk.
- Some women say that the clogging occurs after sleeping in the same position on their side with the bedclothes clumped under their arms, so try to avoid doing this.
- If baby does not nurse well or sleeps through a feeding, express the milk.

Management

- Continue to breastfeed frequently.
- Apply moist, hot compresses before feedings. You can also take a hot shower or soak the affected breast in a sink or bowl of hot water to get the milk flowing.
- Nurse more frequently but for shorter periods of time.
- Massage the affected area toward the nipple during the hot soaks and while nursing.
- Begin each feeding on the affected side.
- Change baby's positions at breast at each feeding to help drain all areas of the breast.

Mastitis

Mastitis is a breast infection. It may occur during the first month following delivery, when baby's nursing is erratic. It often occurs before the letdown reflex is well conditioned. Be aware that mastitis may occur during changes in milk supply and demand. Examples of these changes are times when there are sudden decreases in the number of feedings, when you return to employment, when baby sleeps through the night, or when there is an improper sucking pattern. It also can appear if baby is weaned suddenly, when nursing is abruptly interrupted, when breastfeeding twins, or if a mother becomes run down, overworked, and stressed from trying to do too much (holidays, company, volunteer work, employment, travel, poor nutrition).

Mastitis may occur when cracked nipples are present, often combined with an improper method of hand milk expression.

Mastitis is often caused by a combination of these factors. It is uncomfortable and sometimes painful but it is *not* a cause for weaning or temporarily stopping breastfeeding. In fact, it is even more important that the breast be drained when you have mastitis, because an infection can be the result of an untreated plugged duct.

Signs (may not have all of these)

- Red, hot, sore area on a tender breast.
- Fever greater than 101°F.
- Flu-like symptoms (body aches, headache, fatigue).
- Red streak up the breast and sudden breast pains.

Prevention

- Be sure you are getting enough rest. Do not become overworked or overcommitted trying to be "super mom."
- Nurse frequently and at regular intervals, with the baby in the proper position.
- If you notice plugged ducts or cracked nipples, make sure you treat them promptly.
- Avoid sudden changes or decreases in the number of feedings.

Management

- Go to bed and stay there! Get as much rest as possible, minimizing any household or other commitments. Take the baby to bed with you to make frequent nursings easier.

- Nurse the baby frequently. If baby will not or cannot nurse, use an electric pump or a good hand pump to maintain milk flow.
- Apply hot compresses or soak the affected area in hot water before nursing.
- Take your temperature. Sometimes the temperature rises rapidly with this type of infection. You may feel fine, and an hour later feel like a truck hit you.
- Call your obstetrician, certified nurse midwife, or nurse practitioner. He or she may wish to prescribe an antibiotic to help handle the infection. Follow the directions and take the medication for the full length of time prescribed, even if you start to feel better in twenty-four hours. You do not have to stop nursing if you are on antibiotics.
- Drink plenty of fluids and fruit juices with vitamin C.
- Keep nursing! Your milk is not harmful to your baby, and he will not become infected from drinking it.

By taking good care of yourself, resting, eating nutritious foods, and understanding how breastfeeding works, many of these situations can be avoided or lessened in severity. Following good breastfeeding techniques is your first line of defense against any problems or obstacles that may arise.

BOTTLE FEEDING

There is more to bottle feeding than meets the eye. You will need to decide on the type of formula to use, the bottle, the nipple, and how all of this will be washed or sterilized.

Formula

Most formulas are based on cow's milk that has been extensively modified so that a baby can digest and utilize the nutrients. Because some babies are allergic to or cannot tolerate cow's milk protein, soy-based formulas are also available. Some babies are also allergic to soy formula.

It used to be that there were only a few types of formula to choose from, and before that you had to make your own. Now there are a whole host of liquid and powdered formulas of varying compositions available. They all claim to be closest to mother's milk, so where do you start? The best place to start is to ask your pediatrician or nurse practitioner what they recommend. Formula comes with iron, with low iron, and without iron. Ask about this, too. Often parents keep their baby on the formula they used in the hospital since it seemed to agree with him. This is fine until you realize that the formula in hospitals is given to the hospital at no charge by formula companies. The formula is not really recommended by anyone—it's just what's there at the time. Double check with your own health care provider to see what he recommends.

Types of Formula

Formula comes in prefilled, sterilized, ready-to-feed four-ounce, six-ounce, and eight-ounce bottles. All you need to do with these is to shake them well and put on a nipple. This type of formula is very expensive, and few parents can afford to totally feed a baby this way. They are great for traveling and for middle-of-the-night feedings.

One handy suggestion is to keep the bottle under the covers with you at night so the formula is just the right temperature. Then you don't have to go to the refrigerator and spend time with bottles while a screaming baby waits in the wings.

Ready-to-feed liquid formula also comes in eight-ounce and thirty-two-ounce cans. Shake this, pour it into clean or sterilized bottles, and refrigerate or use within an hour. An opened can should be covered, refrigerated, and used within forty-eight hours.

Concentrated liquid formula comes in thirteen-ounce cans. This concentrated formula must be diluted with water before you feed it to baby. If you use this or leave it with a sitter, make sure that you dilute it exactly as instructed in the directions on the can. The directions are usually in both English and Spanish and include pictures for clarification.

Powdered formula comes in sixteen-ounce cans. It must also be mixed with water before feedings. The powder is thick and the water and formula must be well-shaken to adequately dissolve all the powder. A scoop is included in the can, so do not use any other measures. Formula must be mixed correctly and accurately. Too much or too little is not good for baby. Be precise—this is not your morning coffee! This is the least expensive formula and is often used by mothers who are combining breast- and bottle feeding or who leave a bottle when they go out.

No matter what type of formula you use, make sure to check the date on each can or bottle. All of these products are dated for freshness, just like the products in the grocery store. They do have a limited shelf life. If you do not see a date or if it is coded and you cannot read it, then do not buy it. Do not purchase cans or bottles that are swollen, dented, unlabeled, or damaged in any way.

Wash the top of each can before you open it. Do not buy the thirty-two-ounce cans of formula until your baby is consuming that much in a day. Instead, use the smaller cans. Pour the whole can into bottles and store them in the refrigerator until you need to use them. Prepare enough bottles for twenty-four hours at a time. Always refrigerate opened cans of formula.

Bottles and Nipples

Here, too, there is an amazing amount of equipment to choose from. There are plastic, glass, and disposable bottles. Glass bottles can be easily and thoroughly cleaned, but can break if dropped or thrown. They come in four-ounce and eight-ounce sizes. Plastic bottles come in the same sizes and are either clear or of different colors and shapes. Babies don't care what the bottles look like! Disposable bottles have plastic inner liner bags that the formula goes in and that are thrown away after use. The plastic holder uses a special wide-mouth nipple. Many families use these because they are convenient and require the least amount of energy and time to clean. There are now also completely disposable, one-use bottles and nipples. These can be an expensive way to feed a baby but are convenient for traveling.

You will need eight to ten bottles, eight to ten screw-on rings, and twelve to sixteen nipples if you are not using disposable bottles. Buy the eight-ounce bottles, even though your baby will not take that much at first. It saves you from having to buy more later on.

Bottles and Nipples

Bottles can be glass or plastic. There are disposable bottles which have plastic liners to throw away after use. Bottles usually come in four- and eight-ounce sizes.

Parents should choose bottles and nipples based on what works best for baby. No matter what the advertisers say, no artificial nipple looks like or acts like a human nipple. Baby's suckling action on an artificial nipple will be quite different from the way he will suck on a human nipple. Artificial nipples can be made of rubber or clear silicone. Make sure the nipple has the correct size hole for formula or breast milk. Large nipple openings are for thicker fluids like pulpy juice, or for older babies. Some nipples come in different sizes for younger or older babies. Follow the manufacturer's instructions for cleaning and sterilizing nipples.

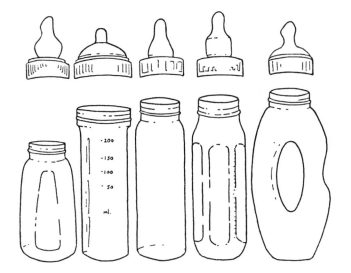

Different types of bottles and nipples. The nipples on the outside left and right are orthodontic; the second nipple is supposed to simulate the breast. The bottle on the far right was developed a few years ago; it is easy for a baby to hold.

There are many different nipples to choose from. The standard nipple is long, made from rubber, and has a hole in the tip. Because of the concern about carcinogens (cancer-causing agents) in the rubber, these nipples are also made from silicone, which is clear in color. Orthodontic nipples are shaped a little differently and are supposed to more closely simulate the contours of a human nipple. The hole is on the top of the nipple and ejects the milk to the roof of the baby's mouth, as it would with breastfeeding. The standard nipple ejects milks to the back of baby's throat, causing him to thrust his tongue forward to control the flow of milk to keep from choking. Orthodontic nipples come in rubber and silicone as well as in a special size for disposable bottles. The nipple that comes with disposable bottles is shorter than the other nipples, and despite the advertising, does not resemble a human nipple. (See the inset on page 51 for more about bottles and nipples.)

The hole in any of these nipples can be of varying size. If your baby chokes and gags when feeding, the hole may be too large. If it takes him forever to feed and he fusses a lot while feeding, then the hole may be too small. The nipple should correspond with the kind of liquid that will be in the bottle. There are four kinds of nipples: one with a cross-cut opening for pulpy juices, and those for formula, milk, and water. You may have to experiment a little to find what's right for your baby.

Bottle and Nipple Care

Ask your pediatrician or nurse practitioner if they recommend sterilizing feeding equipment and for how many weeks or months. Opinions on this vary. Some feel that dishwashers with sani-cycles (high temperature water) are sufficient. Others will advise either what is known as the terminal heating method or the boiling method. (See Table 2.1.) All bottles and nipples must be rinsed after every use and then scrubbed in hot soapy water with a bottle brush and a nipple brush to loosen milk that adheres to the sides. Clean nipple holes with a pin or toothpick and squeeze water through them. If you use disposable bottles the plastic bags are thrown away, but the nipples still need to be scrubbed and boiled or run through the dishwasher.

Table 2.1 Sterilizing Bottles

Terminal Heating Method for Sterilizing Bottles and Preparing Formula	Boiling Method for Sterilizing Bottles
1. Clean bottles, nipples, and rings.	1. Clean bottles, nipples, and rings.
2. Prepare formula and pour into bottles for the day's feedings.	2. Put empty bottles top down in a sterilizer or deep pan with 5 inches of water. Also put in nipples and rings.
3. Place nipples and caps loosely on the bottles.	3. Keep the lid on, and boil 5 minutes.
4. Place in special sterilizer or in three inches of water in a deep pan.	4. Cool and pour in ready-to-feed formula or mix powder or concentrate with boiled water and pour into sterilized bottles.
5. Cover and boil for 25 minutes.	5. Place nipples on bottles and refrigerate.
6. Cool, tighten caps, and place in refrigerator.	

Giving Baby a Bottle

Formula-fed babies generally need somewhere between two-and-a-half to three ounces of formula per day for every pound they weigh. Remember that this is a ball park figure and that all babies differ in their food requirements. You don't have to try to feed them this much at each feeding. Concern yourself more with how much the baby consumes in twenty-four hours. Table 2.2 will give you an idea of daily amounts.

Since every baby's appetite is different and changes constantly, you need to remain flexible and willing to adjust amounts of formula to your baby's requirements.

It is not necessary to heat a bottle of formula on the stove. Breast milk is given to baby at 98.6°F—body temperature. Formula does not need to be any warmer than that. After you take the bottle from the refrigerator, put it under hot running water

Table 2.2.   Typical Daily Amounts of Formula

Baby's Weight	Amount of Formula
6 pounds	15 ounces per 24 hours
7 pounds	17½ ounces per 24 hours
8 pounds	20 ounces per 24 hours
9 pounds	22½ ounces per 24 hours
10 pounds	25 ounces per 24 hours

to take the chill off. *Do not microwave formula!* Because microwaves unevenly heat, it's possible that the bottle will feel cool but actually be boiling hot. There have been several reports in medical literature of babies receiving severe burns in the mouth and throat from microwaved formula.

Each time you feed your baby, sit in a comfortable chair or couch with your back well supported. Support the arm where baby is cradled. Keep his head elevated above his stomach. Always hold your baby close to you. All babies need physical closeness, not matter how they are being fed. Switch baby to the other arm halfway through the feeding after you burp him. This more closely resembles nursing, and helps to properly stimulate and develop both sides of baby's body. Burp baby at the end of each feeding.

Never leave baby unattended with the bottle propped in his mouth! Not only does this practice decrease the attention and contact that baby needs, but it is quite dangerous should baby choke on the formula with no one around. Also, if the bottle is left propped in baby's mouth overnight, it could cause caries (cavities) when baby gets teeth.

When you give your baby a bottle, gently stroke the side of his mouth closest to you. This stimulates the rooting reflex and will cause baby to turn toward your touch and open his mouth. As baby opens up, allow him to draw the nipple far into his mouth. Keep the nipple full of formula by tilting the bottle up. Don't allow baby to suck in lots of air. You may notice that he pauses occasionally in his sucking to both rest and allow a little air back into the bottle so the formula will keep flowing. If the nipple flattens out and baby can't remove formula, break the suction around the nipple while watching for air to bubble in.

How Frequently Will Baby Feed?

Bottle-fed babies can be fed by following the same guidelines that apply to breastfed babies. Feed your baby when he seems hungry. This can be every two or three hours when he is newborn. Stop feeding him when he seems full and the vigorous sucking has stopped. Trying to impose rigid four-hour schedules on little babies is pointless. You don't eat that way; why should he? Baby is used to being continually fed. What does the clock know about how often baby wants food? A young baby's appetite can be very erratic at first. He may want food one-and-a-half hours after his last bottle. Maybe his tummy is not completely empty, but so what? His body tells him it's time for more. He may take three ounces at one feeding and more or less at another. What you are doing is feeding him on demand, letting him take what he needs when he needs it. When you feed him like this you are meeting his needs on his own terms. If you try to stretch out feedings to the magic four hours, you wind up with a crying and sometimes frantic baby. It is easier to give him an ounce or two of formula two hours after his last bottle if he wants it than it is to try and soothe a screaming baby for three hours. After a baby has cried that long, he may fall into an exhausted sleep when finally given the bottle. Then, an hour later, he may wake up and still be hungry. Small, frequent feedings are the norm for new babies. Never force your baby to take the last ounce or drain the bottle if he resists. This practice can result in babies who spit up a lot, are not content, and become very fat and immobile. Excess fat is not good for anyone at any age. Overfeeding is a bad habit to begin. Make sure that other people who feed your baby are aware that he is not to be overfed.

Bottle-fed babies may need a little water occasionally, especially if you notice that your baby's urine is becoming more concentrated. It may take additional water for some babies to handle formula. Do not give fruit juices until your pediatrician or nurse practitioner instructs you to do so. Juices are sometimes recommended if baby becomes constipated from iron-containing formulas.

Do not start solid foods until baby is between four to six months old. Starting solids sooner than this to be the first on the block or to make baby sleep through the night can set up potential allergies in baby, be extremely messy, add excess calories that make him fat, and cause digestive upsets when an immature digestive system tries to tackle something for which it is not yet ready. Some parents even try putting cereal in the formula or using special bottles to feed this mush to their baby. Please do not do this. In the early weeks, using a bottle like this is unnecessary. When baby is ready for solids, using this type of bottle bypasses a normal developmental milestone—that of moving from suckling to a more mature feeding pattern.

COMBINATION FEEDING

Some mothers both breast- and bottle feed their baby for various reasons. This is more common when baby is several months old and mother is returning to school or employment. It is sometimes done earlier if the mother has work commitments, has to be away from baby for long periods of time, or just wishes to do this. It is easier to do if you wait until the milk supply is well established and breastfeeding is proceeding smoothly.

Many babies can handle this with no trouble. Others may get very confused and not feed well until just one method is chosen. Combination feeding will reduce your milk supply, and cause some babies to gradually lose interest in feeding at breast. However, knowing that this is a possibility may help you decide to breastfeed if you are still unsure, and add one more option to your parenting career.

YOUR FEELINGS

New mothers usually feel tired and overwhelmed at first, no matter how they are feeding their baby. This is normal. You have just given birth and assumed a new role in your life. You need to relax and take care of yourself. Get plenty of rest and sleep when the baby does. Talk to other experienced mothers. Our culture does not offer much in the way of education for parenthood. Most of this is learned on the job! Surround yourself with people who support what you are doing. New mothers' groups are a good way to get out of the house with the baby and enjoy the company of other women in the same situation. The confusion, fatigue, and feeling that things are out of control will soon change to confidence and joy in your new role.

Chapter Three

Elimination: What Goes In Must Come Out!

Here is the topic you have all been waiting for! Nothing makes a new father quake in his boots more than the thought of changing dirty diapers! Sometimes the concept of "shared responsibilities" stops with this issue! Actually, it's not as bad as it sounds. You will be doing things that you never thought you would do in a million years or swore that you would avoid at all costs, because this is *your* baby. Wait until it comes time to wipe the runny nose (children seem to have runny noses from birth to age six years). This small part of you is totally dependent on you for his care—care that is given from head to toe. So let's focus on the details that occur about three-quarters of the way down.

MECONIUM

Your baby's first stools are called meconium. This is a black, sticky, odorless substance that is present in the baby's intestines while in the womb. Once she has been born, this stool needs to be eliminated for normal digestion and bowel movements to take place. Most babies pass meconium within the first twenty-four to thirty-six hours after birth.

Fetal waste material is also a reservoir of bilirubin. Increased amounts of bilirubin that the baby can't excrete fast enough will increase and contribute to newborn jaundice. (See pages 8 and 9.) Some studies have shown that the earlier and faster that this meconium is excreted, the less the incidence and severity of jaundice. Breastfeeding encourages rapid passage of meconium, as colostrum (the first food from the breast) acts as a laxative to help expel meconium quickly.

During their stay in the hospital, smart parents usually take a walk together or suddenly need a nap or shower when meconium is first noticed in the diaper. Then the nurse in the nursery gets the job! Sooner or later, however, you will probably get one of these diapers. Washcloths or the wipes used in the hospital and soaked in warm water will usually remove meconium. Sometimes, baby oil on cotton balls is useful for "sticky poop" removal.

By the way, all new parents become stool watchers. You will even find this subject cropping up during polite conversation with other parents. People who do not have children do not understand the emphasis that is placed on stools. They don't realize the amount of time that you spend dealing with this item each day. Nor do they realize that both stools and urine give you clues as to the condition and functioning of your baby.

Once meconium has been eliminated and the baby is receiving breast milk or formula, you will notice what are called "transitional" stools. These transitional stools will change from the black meconium to greenish-brown to a yellowish color with seed-like components if your baby is breastfed, or a brown color if baby is bottle-fed.

BREASTFED STOOLS

As the composition of your breast milk changes from colostrum to true milk, so will the nature of baby's stools. They become soft, semi-liquid or liquid, loose, and seedy in appearance. The color is usually daffodil-yellow with many variations of the shade, and these stools tend to explode from the rectum. The stool has a musty odor that doesn't blow you away when you open the diaper! If the stool gets all over your clothes, Dad, don't panic—it washes out!

The frequency of stooling can range from as often as eight times per day to as frequently as once every few days. Infrequent stooling in a breastfed baby may mean that he needs more time when nursing or needs more feedings. A totally breastfed baby is never constipated. Breast milk is such a perfect food for your baby that it is digested very efficiently and it may take several days for enough fecal material to accumulate to stimulate the bowels to move. Sometimes all you will see is a dark yellow stain.

FORMULA-FED STOOLS

If your baby is being given formula he will also have meconium as his first stool. This will change to a brown-green transitional stool and then to a semi-formed brownish stool with a fairly strong odor. Baby will probably move his bowels two to three times per day.

Formula-fed babies can become constipated. They may have infrequent, hard stools, and show discomfort when trying to pass the stool.

URINE

New babies urinate frequently. Eight to twelve wet diapers in a twenty-four hour period is normal after about five to seven days of age. Before five days or so you will not yet see as many diapers.

Urine should be pale in color and should not have a fishy or foul smell. If the urine is dark yellow or very concentrated, it may mean that baby needs to be breastfed more frequently, or if bottle-fed, he may need water. Baby should be wet at each feeding and probably lots of times in between also.

If your baby is wearing disposable diapers, it is sometimes hard to tell at first if baby is wetting. Most of these diapers are very efficient at drawing the moisture away from the skin and into the padding of the diaper. Because newborns do not pee a lot at one time, you may sometimes need to squeeze the diaper padding to see if baby is wet.

If your baby goes more than six hours without a wet diaper, he may need more fluids. Check with your pediatrician. Baby may be using up more fluid than usual because she is starting a fever or sweating on a hot day.

DIAPERS

One question all new parents ask is, "Should we use a diaper service, disposables, or do our own?" How many years have you gone to school to make this decision? There are no hard and fast rules about this. Whatever you choose will be right for you. Let's talk about each type.

Doing Your Own Diapers

We feel that unless you have live-in help, doing your own diapers during the first weeks is masochistic. The new mother needs to recover from pregnancy and birth. She does not need to spend time at the laundromat or running back and forth to the washing machine, dryer, or outdoor clothes line.

Doing your own diapers involves more than simple washing and drying. Diapers need to be soaked for several hours in a sterilizing solution, washed, and rinsed well to prevent sore bottoms on babies. If ammonia from the urine is still present in the diapers, or if detergents have not been rinsed out completely, diaper rash can be the result. Because of this, diapers need to be rinsed twice, which means you have to reset the washing machine to accomplish this. You can't do the diapers with the rest of your family laundry. Remember also that you can't add colored laundry to diapers in a sterilizing solution because the colors will run.

You will need to purchase about four dozen diapers, plus bleach, sterilizing solution or soaking solutions, and detergent. Baby will be going through about ninety to one hundred diapers a week. The amount will vary. Some parents like to double- or triple-diaper the baby at night to avoid diaper changes in the middle of the night or a sopping wet baby and crib in the morning. Some families use their own diapers at night, and disposables during the day. That way they are not doing as many washes.

When baby is in cloth diapers, he will usually wear plastic pants to keep most of the wet in the diaper. Sometimes baby has extra-sensitive skin and will easily and quickly develop a rash from having moisture trapped so efficiently against his skin. Washable diaper coverings that allow the skin to breathe and release moisture are now on the market. (Many of these will leak, too!) These are somewhat expensive, but seem to help with this problem.

There are all kinds of cloth diapers, from cotton squares that you fold yourself (see the inset on page 66) to shaped, prefolded diapers that do not need folding but take longer to dry, to designer cloth diapers for discriminating bottoms! These diapers are 100 percent cotton. Some cloth diapers have Velcro fastening tapes on them and others will need special diaper safety pins with safety lock heads to prevent baby from being accidentally poked. One brand is constructed with a cotton inner layer against baby's skin and a waterproof outer layer.

Some parents also use what are called diaper liners. These are squares of disposable material that are placed inside washable diapers to keep fluid away from the skin and to trap the worst of the bowel movements, allowing for easier removal from the diaper. Remember parents—the bowel movements have to be placed (somehow) in the toilet before you drop the diaper into the pail to soak. Keep extra disposable diapers around in case of emergency! Many parents who use cloth diapers at home will use disposables when they go out to avoid carrying plastic bags full of dirty diapers. You may or may not find cloth diapers to be more economical.

Some parents prefer 100 percent cotton reusable diapers, because they do not contribute to the increasing problem of solid waste disposal and the product is a natural one. Paper diapers can contain talc, chemically refined paper liners, and petroleum-based plastic. Of course, the plastic pants that go over cloth diapers are also made from petroleum-based plastic. Now, biodegradable disposable diapers are also available.

Diaper Service

Diaper service is sometimes received as a shower gift or chosen to be used during the first few months. The service provides about ninety diapers a week and usually a pail to put them in. They pick up the dirty diapers and deliver a clean bag once a week. The diaper pail that you use should have a deodorizer in it, as the odor after seven days' buildup can be very unpleasant! Parents with diaper service should also keep a couple of boxes of disposable diapers on hand at all times. If you use more than ninety diapers, or if the delivery service is late for some reason, you don't want to be caught short. The costs of diaper services can vary.

Disposable Diapers

These are absorbent paper pads with a plastic outer layer, a middle thicker absorbent layer, and an inner liner designed to draw fluid away from the baby. They do not need pins because they have fastening tapes on them. There are numerous brands on the market, from generic to name brand to Cabbage Patch Kids® in different colors. Some have extra padding in the back or front for girls or boys!

Disposable diapers are truly a convenience product. Some people object to these because of the amount of solid waste they generate, but most parents will use disposables at some time or other. They come in a wide variety of shapes and sizes for different ages and weights, from preemie to toddlers to extra-absorbent overnight sizes. (The ultra absorbent diapers are fine for older babies but aren't necessary for a newborn.) You will probably experiment with different brands until you find your favorite. Some brands come with gathered legs to help keep everything in the diaper and off of you! Many parents appreciate this, especially with the breastfed baby's liquid-type stool! Just make sure that the gathered area is not too tight for baby.

Since it is sometimes hard to tell if your baby is wet when wearing these diapers, you may tear open the tabs only to find that baby is still dry. Buy some masking tape to retape the tabs so you don't waste money. It is best not to use the finger test to check for wetness (putting a finger, sight unseen, into the diaper to check what's there). Some brands of disposable diapers now come with restickable tabs. But restickable tabs lose their stickiness if your fingers are smeared with petroleum jelly or other creams. Most parents go through two or three diapers before they realize this!

Baby will use about ten to twelve of these diapers per day. When you buy these diapers, get the case (four boxes totaling sixty-six diapers). It is much more economical to buy the case at large toy stores or discount/warehouse supermarkets. Buying the smaller box is more expensive. A big case of diapers will last about five-and-a-half days.

Whatever you decide, the diapers you choose to use should fit in with your lifestyle. Even if you don't choose cloth diapers, you should purchase about a dozen of them. These can be used for "burp cloths" (a cloth on your shoulder to catch spit-up milk and a clean place for baby to rest her head). Put one under baby's face and neck while she is sleeping to catch spit-up milk and saliva to keep the sheet clean. They are also your future dusting and polishing cloths!

Changing Diapers

Parents spend a lot of time changing diapers! Life can be made much easier if you have a place set aside where all of your supplies are kept for the changing and dressing routine. You will need a safe, comfortable, and waterproof place to change baby that can easily be cleaned. Most parents purchase, borrow, or are given a changing table, or make or adapt something to suit their needs. Changing tables come in many forms.

One type of table is made of wicker, folds for storage, and has open drawers or shelves for storing diapers and clothing. Other types are made of wood, do not fold up, and also have storage shelves. Some have changing tops that lift up to reveal a plastic bathtub underneath for bathing baby. Newer models have detachable tops, drawers, and pads that later convert to a child's dresser.

Changing areas should have three high sides and wide restraining straps to keep baby from rolling off the top. The table should be at a comfortable height for you to change the baby without having to lean over and strain your back. It should be sturdy, well-balanced, and have a comfortable waterproof pad on which baby can lie. You should have a wastepaper basket, laundry hamper, and diaper pail next to the table.

It is extremely important to *never* leave the baby unattended, even if he is strapped down. Never turn your back or walk away from the table. All of your supplies should be within arm's reach. The phone and doorbell can wait.

Folding Cloth Diapers

You may choose to use cloth diapers. If so, you will need to learn how to fold them so that they are as absorbent as possible. Below are the three most popular ways of folding cloth diapers.

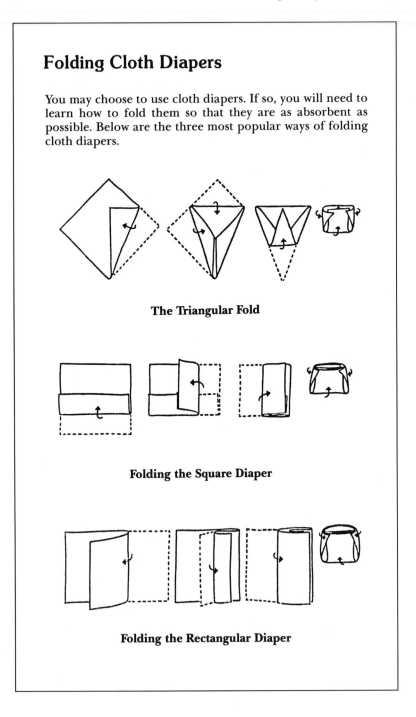

The Triangular Fold

Folding the Square Diaper

Folding the Rectangular Diaper

Diapering Supplies

You do not need a lot of fancy creams, powders, oils, lotions, and potions to apply to a baby's bottom. Clean-up time can be made easy and inexpensive if you use soap and water and cut up squares of old towels.

There are many types of baby wipes on the market. These wipes contain an amazing variety of ingredients guaranteed to clean your baby's bottom better than the competitors. Some parents do not wish to apply all of this stuff, much of which includes perfume and alcohol as main ingredients, ten to fifteen times a day to baby's bottom. These wipes can also get to be quite expensive. (They are convenient, though, when you go out with baby.) Many parents simply cut up old towels into six-by-six inch squares and machine-stitch seam binding around the edges to prevent unraveling. Your true friends will do this for you! Washcloths also do the same job, but most of us do not have fifty washcloths stacked in the linen closet. Washcloths make great baby gifts! Bowel movements are cleaned off with soap and water using the cotton squares. Wet diaper changes usually clean up just fine with warm water on the cloth. Despite claims to the contrary, babies get along just fine without perfumed and greasy bottoms.

When cleaning messy diapers, clean most of the mess with the diaper. Make sure that little girls are cleaned from front to back and that a clean cloth or portion of the cloth is used for each wipe. Rinse with another cloth. Separate all the folds in baby's upper legs and wipe in there, too. Lift baby's bottom up a little by holding both ankles together with one of your fingers be-tween the ankles and raising the legs together toward the head. Wipe baby's backside to complete the cleanup. Dry every skin fold, including the crease between the buttocks. One other help-ful hint—while you are changing a baby boy, keep a diaper draped over his penis. We know many an unwary parent who has experienced not only a drenching shower, but a clean up job that included baby (again), the wall, changing table, changing equipment, and the ceiling! Baby girls can also put forth quite a fountain of urine. Do not lean too close to the area being worked on!

Ointments, creams, and powders are not routinely needed on baby's bottom. Powders can accumulate in skin folds, causing irritation and skin rashes. The powders smell nice but do not contribute to the prevention of diaper rash. Oils, ointments, and creams can function as a moisture barrier, but also seal in moisture if they are applied to skin that is not completely dry. Instead of using creams to prevent diaper rash, change the diaper frequently. If you are using cloth diapers, make sure they are rinsed twice and properly sterilized. Allow baby's bottom to air-dry for a few minutes before putting on a new diaper.

If baby sleeps for long periods during the night, use extra large plastic pants to keep most of the moisture in but still allow air to circulate. If you use plastic pants with side snaps, leave the bottom snaps undone so that the elastic legs do not form a perfect seal. A puddle pad under a sleeping baby reduces laundry loads.

Diaper Rash

Finally, we have a few thoughts on diaper rash. Diaper rash can be anything from slight reddening of the skin to severe inflammation with actual sores on the skin. On baby girls, the labia may be red and sore, and on baby boys, the scrotum can also become irritated. One of the best ways to treat this condition is to change baby's diaper frequently so that he is not in a wet diaper for too long. Clean baby immediately and stay away from creams until the rash is better. The creams prevent air from reaching the skin. Should pustules (fluid-filled sores) or open sores develop, consult your pediatrician. Baby may be quite irritable and fuss frequently when he has a sore bottom. Many babies find that lying on their back or tummy with no diaper on allows them more freedom to kick, which is usually quite enjoyable.

Was all this as bad as you thought?

Remember to remain flexible in the choice of what to use for diapers. All parents have their own reasons for using a particular kind of diaper. Use what works best for you!

Chapter Four
Sleeping

Some parents think that the words "baby" and "sleep" should not be used in the same sentence! We are always amused when mothers- and fathers-to-be declare that their new baby will not cause them to make changes in their life or that they are going to "teach" their baby to sleep though the night early on. Most new parents need to adjust their sleep patterns around the new baby in the early weeks, and sleep or nap when the baby does. Expecting seven to eight hours of uninterrupted sleep every night with a newborn is unrealistic. This chapter will look at sleep needs in the new family.

WHERE SHOULD BABY SLEEP? (SLEEP? WHAT'S SLEEP?)

This question has a couple of answers. Baby can sleep in your room, his own room, out in the hall, in the living room, etc. You must decide what is best for you. Others will tell you the following.

- "The baby should learn to sleep in his own room." (At four days of age?)
- "My baby slept in our room for the first few weeks because it made the night feedings easier."
- "Sometimes all the noises that the baby made kept me up all night, so we put her in a buggy in the hall."
- "Sometimes it was easier just to keep her in bed with me while I was nursing and we would both fall asleep."

Babies do not care where they sleep. They are so smart—
when they are tired, they go to sleep. Any surface will do, from a
padded laundry basket, to a dresser drawer, to a brass crib. It
makes no difference to them!

BASSINET, CRADLE, CRIB—WHICH IS BEST FOR YOU?

A bassinet is sometimes used as a temporary crib until baby is
put into a full-size crib. Bassinets are small and portable. Some
collapse and can be transported in the car. Many are on wheels.
The bassinet can be kept in your bedroom for the first few
weeks.

Many parents who live in a two story home find it convenient
to have the crib upstairs in baby's room and the bassinet down-
stairs where the family's activity is centered. Bassinets and bug-
gies can also be moved out to a porch or into the yard. The
bassinet has a pad, for which you need linens. Baby will quickly
outgrow it, but bassinets are often passed down in families,
borrowed from friends, or found at garage sales. They are also
nice for use in small apartments, as are cradles.

Cradles are also temporary resting places! Many of these are
quite lovely, and some can be hand made using kits that come
with materials and instructions. Cradles also need pads and
linens. Make sure that the cradle is deep enough so that baby
cannot roll out. It should be sturdy and set up so that it is stable
and well-supported.

Cribs come in an amazing variety of styles and colors. Be
aware that whatever type of crib you use, it should conform to
the federal safety standards that require a spacing of not more
than two-and-three-eighths inches between the crib slats. All
metal parts should be smooth; there should be no rough edges.
The latches on the drop side of the crib must be constructed
and placed so that they cannot be accidentally released by baby
from inside the crib, or accidently released by anyone from the
outside.

Make sure that the crib mattress fits properly. If you can fit
more than two fingers between the mattress and the crib, then
the mattress is too small for the crib. Be especially careful of this
if you are using a hand-me-down crib. Measure the width between the crib slats and secure the proper size mattress to avoid

A Safe Crib

Be sure that your baby's crib conforms to federal safety standards. Many older cribs do not.

- The space between the crib rails should no be more than 2⅜ inches (5.9 centimeters). If the rails are wider than this, baby's head could get caught between them.
- The latches that raise and lower the sides of the crib should be placed so that an older baby cannot get to them and accidentally lower them.
- You should not be able to fit more than two fingers between the mattress and the crib.
- The side of the crib, when raised all the way, should be no lower than 22 inches (55 centimeters) above the mattress.
- If the crib is painted, the paint should be nontoxic and lead free.
- There should be no jagged or sharp edges on the crib.

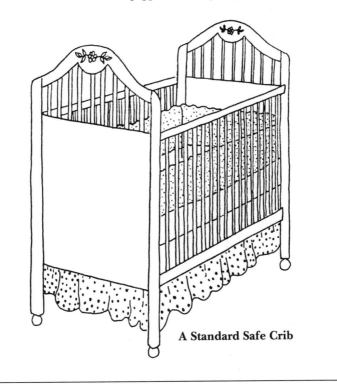

A Standard Safe Crib

accidents. Many older cribs do not conform to the new safety standards.

Full-size cribs have three or four settings so that the height of the mattress can be adjusted. As baby grows, the mattress is lowered. Many cribs can be converted to toddler- and child-size beds so that the one piece of furniture serves for many years.

Many parents will also want to acquire crib bumpers, which go inside the crib. These are vinyl or washable pads that line the crib sides to protect baby's head from the hard crib slats and from drafts. The bumpers are used until baby learns to stand. When that happens, the bumpers, and anything else that would help her climb over the side, are removed from the crib. One other thing about bumpers. Babies love enclosed areas where they seem to feel more secure. Some parents will divide the crib in half with bumpers. One side is a small, snug area for sleep, and the other side can be used as a changing area. Because babies feel more secure in a smaller enclosed area, some parents will use rolled-up towels or small, rolled-up receiving blankets to do the same job as crib bumpers or to make a smaller enclosed space. Boundaries mimic the small space the baby just came from! Parents have often noticed how baby will travel up the crib until his head is resting against the headboard. You can place your baby near the crib bumper to help her feel more secure. Babies do not sleep with pillows.

If you want your baby in your room and your bedroom is big enough, you can place the crib next to the bed at night and lower the crib side next to the bed. Then, if Mom is nursing, she can merely roll over and pull baby toward her and either sit or lie in bed and feed the baby. If you are bottle feeding, consider using the ready-to-feed convenience bottles at night. All you need do with these is place the nipple on the bottle. Who wants to go to the kitchen in the dead of night? Conserve your energy for the first few days you are home.

Some parents find that they cannot sleep well when the baby is in their room. "She is so noisy! We didn't know she would make so many gurgling noises." It is all right to put baby in another room. Don't worry—you will hear her when she needs to eat. If you are really concerned about hearing her cry, or if you have a very quiet or placid baby who does not give loud hunger signals, you might wish to consider using an intercom.

The sending unit can be placed in baby's room and the receiving unit in your room. Some intercoms are battery-operated and some plug into the house electricity.

SLEEPING PATTERNS

Most healthy, full-term newborn babies are wide awake and alert for an hour or so following their birth. They will often sleep rather soundly for about a day or so after that, and then start looking around for food!

Babies' sleep patterns are very erratic. They do not sleep the way adults do. Some babies spend much time asleep—up to eighteen to twenty hours (but not all in a row!). Other babies do not want to miss anything and spend a remarkable amount of time awake or half-awake. You may notice that your baby drifts from sleep to wakefulness very gradually, so that you are not always sure if he is awake or asleep. It is typical to see a baby begin a feeding wide awake and ravenously hungry, only to suck a few times and drift off into blissful sleep, interrupted now and then by short periods of sucking. Soon he drifts off into sound sleep where nothing will wake him. This is very common, as is the baby who just cat naps for twenty minutes at a time around the clock! Remember that babies have no watches. They do not know, nor do they care, about night and day. They respond to basic physiologic needs, not routines and schedules.

Many babies will take a five-hour sleep stretch. During the first few weeks, this might occur during the day rather than at night. The reason they sleep more during the day may be related to their sleep/wake cycle while they were still *in utero*. When did your baby wake when you were pregnant? Didn't you get kicked during the 11 p.m. news, or right after you climbed into bed and relaxed? You rocked baby all day while you worked. No wonder he wakes up at night! We recommend that, for the first few days, you wake baby during the day, if necessary, to feed him. This may help him to adjust to sleeping longer at night. Feeding baby frequently during the day may help with the message that nighttime is for sleeping. Night feedings should be on demand—do not skip them. Don't let your baby sleep longer than six hours without being fed. This goes for both bottle- and breastfed babies.

These erratic sleeping patterns can be difficult for parents. There is nothing that you can do to *make* a baby sleep. Some babies will sleep all day and then be bright-eyed and ready to play after the 2 a.m. feeding! Trying to schedule sleeping is just as fruitless as trying to schedule hunger, going to the bathroom, or the sunrise!

Listed below are a few hints that will help you cope during this period of time.

- Place baby in his crib at night so that he comes to associate the crib with when he is really sleepy. Bring him out with the rest of the family when he is awake so that he associates wakefulness with company. *Babies should not spend long periods of time isolated in a crib.*

- When baby is sleeping you do not need to whisper and tiptoe around the house. The normal noise level of the house will usually not disturb a baby at this age. They learn to tune out when they are tired. If you enforce a soundless household when baby is sleeping, you may find that there comes a time when that is the only way baby will be able to sleep, and this may continue as he grows older. Some parents leave on a radio or play soft music to provide background noise while they go about their business.

- When your baby wakes at night, be sure that he is really awake before you pick him up. Many times a baby will wake or just stir a bit, make some noises, and go back to sleep. If you pick him up at this point, he may eat, but not very efficiently. When you put him back he may think, "Oh, was I hungry?" and then really wake up about thirty minutes later. When baby stirs, wait a few minutes and see what happens. If he is really hungry he will not go back to sleep. Make sure, however, that you do not wait too long, because a ravenous baby may not want to go back to sleep after being awake.

- Some parents will help baby find his fist or thumb to suck on during the night. They feel that this helps the baby learn some self-comforting measures so he can get back to sleep by himself.

- Gather all the equipment or supplies that you might need during the middle of the night so that you do not spend more time awake than is really necessary. As we mentioned before, if you are bottle feeding, try using ready-to-feed bottles for night feedings. Have two bottles and nipples by your bed so you do not need to make a trip to the refrigerator. You do not need to warm the bottle in the middle of the night, as this type of bottle will already be at room temperature, which is just fine for baby. We know one couple who kept the bottle under the covers so it would be at body temperature when baby awoke.

Breastfeeding mothers are often thirsty at night. Put a pitcher of ice water by the bed. When baby wakes up, the ice will be melted and the water comfortably cool. If a warm drink helps you get back to sleep, keep it in a thermos bottle by your bed.

- Some parents find that their baby has a difficult time going back to sleep in the middle of the night (or any other time, for that matter!). They have found a wonderful piece of equipment called the baby swing. Some of these swings come with seats that recline, and others actually have a cradle that swings. The motion is often helpful in lulling baby to sleep. The older models have very noisy cranks that often awaken baby and half the neighborhood when they are wound up. Most of the newer ones operate much more quietly. Some are battery-operated and run for many hours.

- One of the fastest ways to get baby back to sleep in the middle of the night is to bring him into bed with you. Your heartbeat, and the warmth he feels when he is held close to your body, are very soothing.

- Usually what disturbs a baby most and wakes him up are internal activities—hunger, cold, pain, etc. If you are putting baby to bed for the night, take some extra time to make him comfortable by following the suggestions below.

—Feed baby right before *you* go to bed.

—Take a few extra minutes to finish burping him.

—Some parents wrap baby very securely (like he was in the hospital) so that his own movements do not fully awaken him.

—Place baby on her tummy or propped on her side to that she does not choke on spit-up milk. To prop baby on her side, place a rolled-up receiving blanket behind her. This is often done in the hospital, as the baby is often kept in this position until the umbilical stump falls off.

—Dim or darken the room so that if baby wakes she will not be encouraged to remain awake watching her toys or mobiles.

—Leave a fifteen-watt night light on in baby's room so that if you need to attend to him at night you will not have to turn on the bright overhead light.

—If baby is in cloth diapers, put three diapers on him at night so he will not awaken early because he is soaking wet. This eliminates the need for changing diapers in the dead of night, which will often bring a baby to full alertness.

—When you pick up baby to feed her in colder weather, place an electric heating pad (on the warm or medium setting) or a heavy blanket in baby's crib. When the feeding session is done, remove the heating pad or blanket from the crib and put baby back. This avoids "transition waking," which means that baby is asleep in your arms, but as soon as you put her in her crib, she wakes up.

Think about this—when you get up to go to the bathroom on a cold night, doesn't it take you a while to get back to sleep after you hit those cold sheets? Another technique that sometimes helps with this type of waking is to feed the baby on a mattress that you have put on the floor. If you are nursing, lie on your side so that when you are done you can place your baby on her tummy, which is very close to the position in which you were nursing her. Bottle feeding mothers can do the same thing.

—Soothing background music may encourage baby to go back to sleep if she wakes early.

SLEEPING THROUGH THE NIGHT

"Sleeping through the night"—fact or fantasy! This depends on how you define "sleeping through the night." Picture this: Two mothers are talking. They both have five-week-old babies.

Mom #1: "My baby sleeps through the night. Does yours?"

Mom #2: (Thinks to herself, "Mine is up every four hours at night.") "No, not yet."

Mom #1: "Oh, that's too bad." (Gloating! New parents can be very competitive.)

Mom #2: Thinks, "Oh, my—what am I doing wrong?" (Goes back home and reads the books!)

What did you detect from this scene, besides competition? Mom #2 should have asked Mom #1 how she defines "sleeping through the night." Instead, she assumed that they both had the same understanding of this term. She may have been relieved to hear that for many parents sleeping through the night means midnight to 5 a.m.! We define sleeping through the night as 8 p.m. to 8 a.m.! We know parents of third and fourth graders who haven't seen their children do this yet!

One of the scariest events in your new lives as parents is the first morning you awake before your baby! Talk about panic! You jump out of bed in a cold sweat, only to find your little babe still sawing z's, in a deep sleep. He's getting older! Just remember though—if your baby sleeps for long periods of time at night, he will probably want and need to eat very frequently for a few feedings—every one-and-a-half to three hours—to make up for lost time.

One last thought about sleeping. Many people judge how good or bad a baby is by how long he sleeps. There is no such thing as a bad baby. Why shouldn't the sleep patterns of a baby be just as varied as adults'? Don't you know night owls and early birds, people who need lots of sleep and people who need little? Variations in sleep requirements are part of what makes your baby special. Respect nature and allow baby his individuality. You cannot control his sleep, only the environment that allows him to get the amount of sleep that he needs.

Chapter Five

Crying: A Means of Communication

Why do babies cry? Infants cry as a means of communication. Babies rely on crying to make contact with Mom and Dad or anyone else within earshot! As baby grows older crying is replaced with speech.

What upsets and comforts a newborn changes as she develops. What upsets and comforts one baby will not necessarily upset or comfort another infant. All babies are individuals right from birth, and they are all different in the way they cope with life outside the womb. Babies may cry because they are hungry, wet, uncomfortable, or in pain, cold, bored, frustrated, lonely, or have been sitting in the infant seat too long and need a change of scenery. Have you heard people tell you that you will quickly learn why your baby is crying? Well, don't count on it! Most parents can distinguish between three different *patterns* of crying, not necessarily *why* the baby is crying or what will soothe her. The three patterns are:

1. A "standard" cry that tells of some need. It starts intermittently and at a low intensity and gradually becomes louder and more rhythmical.
2. The "angry" cry. This is a louder, more insistent version of the "standard" cry.
3. The pain or distress cry. This starts suddenly and loudly and is followed by a short silence (breath holding) and then short, gasping cries. This type of crying may cause the parents to run to the baby and emit short gasps too!

Interpreting crying requires skills that come with your growth and development as parents. Most parents do not base their interpretation of crying on the differences between the sounds themselves. They start to rely on other things to help them decide how to respond to the cries. These other features may be how long it has been since the last feeding, how well baby fed last time, how restless he has been, when he last slept and for how long, or how easy he is to soothe.

How you respond to your crying baby is also dependent on your feelings about "spoiling" a child. In the first few days, every time your baby cried you picked her up, and she nestled into your chest as if to say, "Oh, thanks Mom or Dad. I got real scared. I couldn't hear a heartbeat. I'm glad to be back home." The baby has been carried and rocked by another human being for nine months. We don't know why parents expect babies to be content in a plastic bassinet! The idea that picking up a crying infant will reward the crying and teach her to do it more often is a common one, and you will hear it all the time. "Don't pick her up all the time, you'll spoil her." Now think about that piece of advice. Does it feel right? Don't you wish that someone would hold *you* when you cry? Pick up that child! It's *your* baby and *you* should do what feels good. You cannot spoil a baby at this age. You are teaching your baby trust when you respond to her needs. The outside world is crazy enough!

Recent studies on crying and comforting have shown that the more attention a child gets in the first year, the less demanding she will be at age two or three. By letting a young baby "cry it out," parents may really be teaching the child that in order to get someone to respond to her needs, she must cry increasingly louder and longer to get results. This is exactly the opposite of what parents and children really want.

CAUSES OF CRYING AND COMFORTING TECHNIQUES

Hunger is probably the most common cause of crying. If it is really hunger that is causing baby to cry, then only breast milk or formula will stop the crying. Pacifiers or water will not do the trick.

If you are breastfeeding, you will notice that breastfed babies require frequent feedings. These babies will usually need to be fed about every two or three hours or on demand, whichever comes first. This phrase is important. Most babies loudly announce their wish for food! Some babies, however, do not give clear signals for when they are hungry, and do not cry to be fed. They may make only small noises, or simply awaken and lie there. People may tell you how "good" your baby is, but make sure that he is fed just as frequently as his noisy neighbor.

Studies have shown that nursing mothers who feed their babies frequently and do not try to extend the times between feedings or impose rigid feeding schedules on their babies have babies who cry less. Breastfed babies require about eight to twelve feedings in twenty-four hours and about fifteen to twenty minutes on each breast at each feeding. You may also notice that between seven to ten days of age, at six weeks, and at about three to six months of age, your baby will experience a "growth spurt." This is usually loudly announced by your baby as he makes constant requests for food. These increased bouts of crying and fretfulness may have you baffled as to their cause. Your baby is telling you that he is growing and needs more food. The more you nurse him, the more milk you will make. This is the law of supply and demand! Short, frequent feedings (ten minutes on each side every one-and-a-half to three hours), are far better than long, infrequent ones (twenty to thirty minutes on each side every four hours). Young babies have very erratic hunger patterns. If your baby is crying loudly, offer the breast and see if this helps, even if it has only been one-and-a-half hours since the last feeding.

Bottle-fed babies also experience growth spurts. Do you only eat at four-hour intervals? Don't you snack occasionally? Many parents of young babies are surprised that these little people eat so often during twenty-four hours. Breast milk is digested and used rapidly by a baby. Babies have small tummies that are not designed to hold seventeen pounds of food at a feeding. Babies are also social creatures and have a need for social contact. A great deal of this interaction comes at feeding time. When there are ten or twelve feeding times during the day, there are many opportunities that encourage close contact with Mom and Dad! "But," you say, "I don't eat that often." Oh really? Let's see. Breakfast, 10 a.m. coffee break, lunch, 3 p.m. snack, 5 or 6 p.m. appetizer, dinner, evening popcorn in front of T.V., and midnight snack. That makes eight times!

With formula-fed infants, parents should be concerned more with the total number of ounces the baby consumes in twenty-four hours, not with the amount of ounces consumed at each feeding. Your baby may have one ounce at one feeding and at the next consume five ounces! Check with your pediatrician or nurse practitioner regarding the recommended ounces per day for your individual baby.

It is not a wise idea to force baby to consume everything in the bottle. This contributes to spitting up and fat babies. Baby's appetite varies and should be respected.

Another thing to remember when bottle feeding: *Never* prop up the bottle in baby's mouth and leave the room. This prevents the close contact that baby needs and can be dangerous should baby choke.

If you attempt to keep baby on a strict four-hour feeding schedule, you may find yourselves in a miserable situation. The baby will wake up and cry. As you try to hold him off because the clock says it "isn't time" he cries more, and you become exhausted, when all he really wants is food. You can't feel his hunger, and the clock can't regulate it, but he knows when he is hungry! Nothing you do will really soothe him until you feed him.

After a session like the one described above, it is not uncommon to see an exhausted baby who does not suck or feed well. He may take only an ounce or two, fall into an exhausted sleep, and wake in an hour to start all over again. In her book, *Your Baby and Child From Birth to Age Five*, Penelope Leach says,

> So don't fall into the trap of thinking that if you feed your baby whenever he seems hungry he will get into the habit of demanding food frequently. He does not wake from habit, he wakes from hunger. When he is mature enough not to be hungry so often he will not wake up and cry.

Many babies fret for food even when they are gaining weight normally. They are usually being rigidly fed only a certain amount at a certain time. This takes care of baby's overall food requirements but does not take into account his current appetite during the growth spurt. If you feed your baby when he is hungry, he will take the "required" number of ounces with less crying.

PACIFIERS

You have now nursed or bottle fed your baby, yet he is still cranky and sucking his fists. Now what? (Isn't this fun playing trial and error!?)

What about a pacifier or thumb? Maybe your reaction to this is, "I don't want my baby using a pacifier. I hate those plugs hanging out of kids' mouths at the shopping mall!" Or, "I don't want my baby sucking his thumb—he'll get buck teeth!" Well, hang on. Your baby was sucking his fingers *in utero* way before

Choosing a Pacifier

If you decide to give your baby a pacifier, make sure that you use one that will not come apart—baby may choke if it breaks into pieces. The pacifier should be a one-piece unit. Pacifiers come in different sizes for babies of different ages. Two kinds of pacifiers appear below.

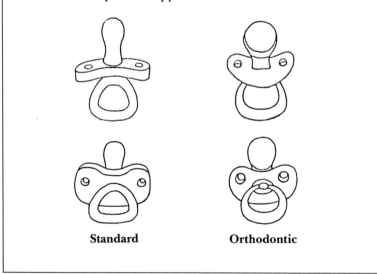

Standard   Orthodontic

you met him. All babies love to suck. It is a feeding reflex and provides comfort and security. Some babies are even born with a blister on their thumb from sucking it before they were born! There is really nothing wrong with pacifiers or thumbs when they are used to meet the sucking needs of infants after they have been fed. Pacifiers become problems when adults use them as plugs! There can be a real control struggle at about three years of age when Mom and Dad say to their child, "Get that pacifier out of your mouth." "I'll put mustard on that thumb." "You can't go to nursery school with a pacifier." Have you already heard these lines? So now the three year old looks up at his parents as if to say, "I'll suck this pacifier until I'm fifty." The control issue arises, and guess who's going to win!

Sucking on a pacifier has a definite effect on babies. It relaxes movements of the stomach, intestines, and major muscles. The sucking is rhythmic and baby's thrashing about is reduced. But a pacifier should never be used in place of feeding or parental attention, and a baby who does not breastfeed well should not be given a pacifier. Each baby's need to suck varies; those with a strong desire to suck will do well using a pacifier.

If you choose to use a pacifier, you may need to teach your baby how to use it. Many infants tongue thrust (push their tongue forward when an object is put in their mouth). This shoots the pacifier across the room! When you find a pacifier that baby likes, buy a few of that brand so you always have a spare, especially at 2 a.m.! Dads can often catch a quick nap by lying on the couch with baby on his chest, holding the pacifier in baby's mouth. This way of handling a pacifier ensures that the pacifier is not used as a substitute for parenting and contact. Pacifiers should be sturdy and unable to come apart. A pacifier should *not* be secured to baby by tying it around her neck! Tie the pacifier through a buttonhole in baby's sweater or to the side of the stroller to keep it from falling on the floor.

IS IT COLIC?

Every time that your baby cries does someone come up and tell you he has colic? Do they say that word in the same tone of voice as if they were referring to bubonic plague? What is this mysterious malady that stalks infants and new parents?

Well, colic is not a disease. Experts disagree on just what colic is, but many point out that it is probably a combination of factors that cause baby to cry so much. Many babies cry a lot during the early weeks of life. An average two or three hours of crying per day is not unusual. Some babies cry more, some less. Colic is often characterized by some or all of the following.

- Nonstop crying spells during which baby cannot be comforted. If anything works, it is usually for a short period of time only. This is the part that drives parents crazy!
- No illness in the baby. These babies are healthy and no disease process or physical cause for the crying can be found.
- A large amount of crying that occurs repeatedly. More than three hours a day of crying may be a clue to this. However, all babies have good days and bad days. Colic is like that, too. It can come and go.
- Crying, as described above, that starts at about two or three weeks of age and lasts to about four months of age.
- Somewhat predictable periods of time during the day when the intense crying occurs. This is typically from late afternoon until 10–11 p.m. This varies, though!

Colic probably occurs in about 20 percent of babies and is seen in all cultures. Defining the difference between normal crying and colic is not always easy. You must remember that a great many infants will have fussy spells in the early evening.

Many parents say that their colicky babies have quick mood changes, are easily startled, do not adapt well to new events or people, and are gassy, with legs drawn up and fists clenched during crying spells. They are also easily awakened and squirmy. Some parents call their babies "difficult" babies. In his book, *Crybabies Coping With Colic: What to do When Baby Won't Stop Crying,* Dr. Marc Weissbluth suggests that colic is part of a relationship between the following.

- Increased amounts of crying.
- An infant who responds dramatically to small changes in his environment.
- An infant who has difficulty sleeping.

- An infant who is described as having a difficult temperament.

He also suggests that there are probably several physiological disturbances that could cause colic. Some people suggest that these babies have gas that is difficult for them to expel.

A DEEP, DARK SECRET

What if the baby swing has been click-clacking for hours and your little angel is still howling? You may be absolutely astounded at your next response. You may walk up to your crying baby and shout, "Shut up!"

What is happening to you? Where is your control? Why are you shouting at a three-week-old baby? Some parents have even picked up the baby, looked her in the eye, and said, "If you don't stop crying, you will never have any brothers or sisters!" Or maybe a thought flashed through your mind—"Maybe I'll just leave her here and go out for a long walk all by myself." This is your emotional (not intellectual) side coming through. Maybe all of a sudden you had a thought about squeezing her tightly to quiet her. This thought puts you at a complete and sudden standstill. "Oh my goodness," you think, "I could be a child abuser. What has happened to me? We waited eight years to have this baby and I can't even take care of her."

The new mother calls the new father at work: "Honey, the baby has been crying for so long and I just had a feeling that I wanted to throw her away. You'd better come home—I'm losing my mind!" New father thinks, "Oh, no, she really sounds upset. I'd better get home." He arrives home to find new mother sitting on the couch in the fetal position, sobbing and sucking her thumb. She figures the police and social worker are outside the door, waiting to take her away for child abuse.

You are not a child abuser just because you had a thought! Thought is a long way from deed. Call a friend who has an older child. Ask her if she ever felt that way. If she is honest she'll tell you that she can distinctly remember the day when she thought that she was the most horrible mother in the world. No one ever tells mothers that they are allowed to be human, so they go around feeling guilty all the time.

This is one of those deep, dark secrets that no one wants to talk about. Who wants other people to know that they had these thoughts? What this feeling should do is alert you to the fact that you will never be all things to all people! But to be able to take care of someone else, you must first take care of yourself.

Let's go back to the moment when you felt that you were losing control. What were you upset with? The crying, right? Not the baby. You were angry with the behavior, not the person. You see, you can only guide and direct behavior. You will never control your child in all ways. There is a gift you can give your baby that he will carry for the rest of her life. That gift is self-esteem. It does not come in a box from the toy store. It is a feeling about one's self that starts to be nurtured at birth. You love your baby always, but his behavior may be trying at times. When he is a toddler, it will be harder work to respond to this type of behavior. An example: "I love you honey, but I don't like the fact that you just knocked over all the plants in the family room."

Crying varies from day to day, and what comforts a baby differs from hour to hour! Whatever is the cause of your baby's crying, the following suggestions may be helpful in soothing him.

- Motion or rocking is usually more effective than just being propped up in an infant seat. Motions that are helpful include:

  —Picking him up and holding him over your shoulder.
  —Rocking him in a cradle, swing, or rocking chair.
  —Pushing him in a baby carriage or stroller.
  —Carrying baby in a front pack baby carrier.
  —Taking him for automobile rides.
  —Massaging him.
  —Swaddling or gently wrapping him.

- More soothing techniques include singing, humming, music, and running the vacuum cleaner (don't really vacuum— you'll wear yourself and the carpeting out!).
- Some people even place baby in an infant seat on top of the washer or dryer when it is running. But you must make sure that someone is there to prevent baby from vibrating off the

machine and onto the floor!

- Baby may calm down when he watches a playful mobile, television, or fish swimming in a fish tank.
- It may soothe baby to suck on a pacifier, his thumb, or your finger.
- You may try keeping the room dim and quiet.
- Sometimes doing nothing will decrease the amount of stimuli that may be aggravating the situation. Overstimulation is sometimes a cause of crying.
- Baby may like warmth on his stomach; try a warm water bottle.
- Medications usually do not help, but you need to check with your pediatrician. Home remedies should *not* be given without the approval of your pediatrician.
- Try giving baby a warm bath, or take him into the tub with you.
- Accept and love your baby, even with all the crying. This baby needs as many hugs and kisses as his quiet cousin.

Give each of these techniques that you try a couple of days to see if they work. Don't run through this list in an hour and say that you have tried everything and nothing works! Try combinations of techniques. Remember that what worked on Monday may not work on Wednesday.

If your baby has colic, remember that colic is not caused by anything you thought or did during your pregnancy, labor, or delivery. It is not your fault. Its cause is unknown. Colicky babies are healthy and do very well once they are a little older.

Remember, colic is self-limiting. It will pass by the time your baby is three or four months old. You may not see the light at the end of the tunnel, but it's there!

Parents sometimes need a break. Get relief for yourself by getting away from your baby. Sometimes the best thing you can do is to take yourself out of the situation so that when you return you will be refreshed and more effective.

Hire two teenagers (to help each other), a college student, a Girl Scout (they can earn badges by doing this), a senior citizen, a friend, or a relative to watch baby while you go out, go to sleep, or get something done around the house. Check out local baby sitting co-ops. These are groups of parents who babysit for each other. There are usually many parents in this type of group who are not intimidated by a crying baby.

Don't isolate yourself from the rest of the world. Sometimes the most helpful resources are other parents with fussy or colicky babies. Start a play group, or join an already existing one, or a discussion group, to help gain a new perspective. Take lessons or classes to make sure that you get out of the house.

Remember that all babies cry during the dinner hour. Get someone to look after baby during this time so that you're assured of one peaceful time during the day, and have this as a goal to work toward.

If you can, schedule any pediatrician visits for as late in the afternoon as possible or for evening hours. This may help your pediatrician evaluate your baby's crying and prove to yourself that the problem really exists! There is nothing worse than going to see your pediatrician or nurse practitioner at 10 a.m. with a sweet, smiling baby while you describe wild screaming sessions!

Keep a diary of baby's behavior and amount of crying time. It may seem like baby cries all day, but looking at the diary may help put the crying in perspective.

Mothers should make sure they get enough rest. This is not easy, but your ability to cope decreases as your fatigue increases. It is important to try and have confidence in yourself as a parent, and to develop a sense of humor. Focus on all the good and happy parts of your baby and of being a parent. It's easy to get lost and overwhelmed by the 25 percent of the day when baby is crying.

Just as you have to accept your own humanness, you have to accept the humanness of those you live with, including your beautiful new baby. What about the man or women that you live with? Doesn't he or she have certain behaviors that you can't control? Accept your humanness!

Chapter Six
Baby's Bath

At some point while you are in the hospital you will be shown how to bathe your baby. If you had your baby in an alternative birthing center or at home, a nurse will usually demonstrate this or help you at home. It doesn't matter when or where you were shown how to bathe your baby. Most of the instruction you receive is very hard to apply when you actually begin to bathe the baby! The first time you try, you may forget where to start or in which direction to proceed. This chapter will help you become acquainted with, and be organized for, the bath.

Until the umbilical cord stump falls off, you will not be immersing baby in a tub of water—a sponge bath is usually sufficient.

The purpose of bathing is to remove dry skin, oils, and dust. Since there are no rules, it is up to you when and how you bathe your baby. As we have already mentioned, you should be cleaning the baby's genital area frequently, as well as washing the face and neck about once a day. As far as tub baths are concerned, it depends on the weather. In the winter, probably three or four times a week is sufficient. In the summer, maybe daily. Babies sweat just as adults do, and baths help keep them cool in the heat. As your baby grows, baths often become daily events because he is having large bowel movements or is waking from naps or a long night's sleep totally saturated.

It does not matter whether you bathe baby in the morning, afternoon, or evening. Do whatever is easiest in your home. Some fathers like to do the bathing in the early evening. Other fathers will do everything else *but* that, as they are uncomfortable with a slippery newborn. Some babies settle better and sleep longer following a bath. If this is the case, why have baby sleep half the day after a morning bath? An evening bath may help quiet a fussy baby.

It is wise to bathe the baby in a warm area; perhaps the kitchen after dinner, when the area has been warmed from the oven. Some parents choose to use a small bathroom that can be easily warmed by running a hot shower for a few minutes.

You may find that the first few baths are rather nerve-wracking. Wet, soapy babies are slippery and usually squirm and scream. You may wonder if it is really worth it and whether it will always be like this. As the baby gets older and is able to sit unassisted, baths become fun times. For right now, most parents find it easier to manage the bath by using a small, special baby tub made of molded plastic. Some of these tubs fit right into the sink, while others are designed for use on a table or countertop. The tubs come in different sizes and, because baby grows quickly, you may want the larger version.

To make bathing even easier, many parents use sponge-like cushions that fit into a small tub, a regular tub, or a sink. These sponges are molded to fit baby's contours and hold him in one place with his head above the water. The baby tub can also be placed in the regular tub, although it might be a strain on your back to lean over to bathe the baby. You can also simply bring the baby into the bathtub with you, and both take a relaxing bath while snuggled together! Babies love this!

If you are bathing baby in the sink or tub, keep him away from faucets. Hot water from the spigot can easily burn a young baby. There are also foam covers for the faucet to keep baby from bumping his head.

When your baby can sit up and is ready for more water play, you can use another piece of equipment called a tub ring. This is a molded plastic circle suspended on four legs that attach by suction cups to the bottom of the tub. This tub rings frees your hands for washing, shampooing, and playing with rubber duckies and other bath toys!

The most important thing to remember about bathing baby is to *never* leave her alone in the tub, even for a minute. It takes only a few seconds for a baby to slip, inhale water, or grab the hot water faucet.

Make sure that you have all your supplies at hand before you start the bath. Organization is the key. If the phone rings, you can either ignore it or take the baby with you while you answer it. (Cordless phones eliminate this problem!)

A great bathing technique is to fill the big tub with warm water and have Daddy climb in first. Mom then hands in the baby. They can have a good time playing with the toys while Mom goes out! Some mothers take a midday relaxation bath with baby. Mom puts the infant seat next to the tub, lines it with a thick towel, undresses, and wraps the baby in the towel. Then she gets into the tub, picks up the baby, washes her, relaxes snuggled next to baby, places baby back in the infant seat wrapped in the towel, and leans back and relaxes for awhile.

You may have been given a baby bath demonstration in the hospital. If you forgot everything, use the list below and the illustrations on page 95 as a guide.

WHAT YOU WILL NEED

Collect everything that you need for your baby's bath. Supplies can include the following.

- Baby tub, or several towels on a countertop or table if baby is not yet ready for a tub bath.
- Sponge insert for the tub (if you have one).
- Towel on bottom of the sink if you are using a sink.
- Warm (not hot) water.
- Four cotton balls.
- Baby shampoo.
- Baby soap (Castile soap, or mild facial soap minus the deodorants and perfumes).
- Two washcloths.
- Two towels—one small, one large.
- Diaper.
- Baby clothes.
- Oils, lotions, and powders are *not* routinely necessary.

WASHING BABY'S FACE AND HAIR

You will bathe baby by starting from the cleanest area and finishing with the dirtiest. Baby's face and hair may be washed before you undress him or you can undress baby but keep him wrapped in a towel to prevent chilling.

Moisten one cotton ball and squeeze out the excess water. This will be used to clean one eye, wiping from the inner part of the eye (near the nose) to the outer part. Moisten the other cotton ball and gently wipe the other eye. The other two cotton balls can be used to wipe the outer ear. (Do not insert cotton swabs into baby's ears or nose.) Baby's face can then be sponged off with a moistened washcloth. Lift up the chin and wipe under the neck, too.

Holding the baby in the "football" hold, wet the baby's scalp using your cupped hand. Apply a small amount of shampoo and gently rub all over the scalp. Talk soothingly to baby, as he may not be fond of getting his hair washed. This is one thing that doesn't change with age! All kids hate having their hair washed! Using your cupped hand, rinse out all the shampoo. Do not put baby's head under the water spout! Dry baby's scalp with the small towel.

SPONGE BATH BEFORE CORD FALLS OFF

If the umbilical cord stump has not yet fallen off, you will give your baby a sponge bath after cleansing his face and scalp.

Place baby on a towel or pad with a towel over it. Keep the parts of baby covered that are not being bathed. Moisten the washcloth, put soap on it, and wash the baby's chest, abdomen, and back. Rinse off the soap, pat dry, and cover that part of baby. Next, soap the front and back of baby's legs, making sure to get into all the folds and creases. Pat dry, taking special care to separate and dry the creases. Then, soap again and clean the genitals, making sure to wipe from front to back on girls. On little boys, remember to wash and dry under the scrotum.

Place baby on a dry towel or pad and dress him. Some parents like hooded towels, as they keep baby's head warm.

TUB BATH

A tub bath proceeds the same way as a sponge bath except that you don't cover the baby as you go. If you have a sponge insert to support the baby in the tub, this leaves both hands free for

Bathing Your Newborn

Make sure you have every-
thing you need for your baby's bath before you begin
bathing him. If you are giving
baby a sponge bath, use the
football hold and gently wet
his hair using water from
your cupped hand. Don't put
your baby's head under the
faucet!

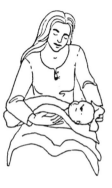

If you are giving him a
bath in a small tub, be sure to
keep one hand and arm be-
hind baby's head and shoulders, as illustrated.

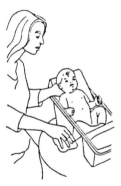

To lift him out, keep one
hand behind his head and
shoulders, and place the
other under his bottom. As
soon as you remove him from
the tub, wrap him in a soft,
dry towel and pat him dry.

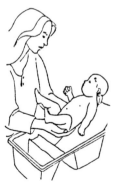

washing. Just be sure that you keep a hand near baby should he decide to try out for the Olympic diving team! If you do not have this sponge insert, one hand must be kept behind baby's head and shoulder, gripping under one of baby's arms to prevent baby from slipping under water. These early baths are often two-adult projects!

Although it may seem a little complicated at first, you will soon become accustomed to bathing your baby. You may even enjoy it!

Chapter Seven

Baby's Health and Health Care

Many decisions and plans are made during pregnancy and the early weeks after your baby is born. Although you have a lot on your mind, like diapers, cribs, and the whole idea of being a parent, take some time to think about health care for your baby. You have an obstetrician or midwife for your pregnancy, and a dentist for your teeth. You will also need a doctor for your baby. Most parents take their children to a pediatrician, a physician whose specialty is children. Some parents use the services of a general or family physician who specializes in taking care of the whole family. Physicians can be found in private practice, either alone or as a group. They may also practice in a clinic, a Health Maintenance Organization or other prepaid health plan, a hospital, or a neighborhood health center. There are many physicians out there, but which one is right for you? The following section will help you find and evaluate a physician for your child.

FINDING AND CHOOSING A PEDIATRICIAN

Ideally, you will choose a pediatrician before baby is born. This will give you plenty of time to find a physician, as well as allow you to contact more than one for comparison. Choosing a doctor early also has another advantage. Should a problem arise with your pregnancy that may affect the baby as a newborn, both obstetrician and pediatrician can discuss this in advance of the delivery. When you are admitted into the hospital or birthing center, your nurse will ask you for the name of your pediatrician. The hospital will call the pediatrician after the baby is born. Generally, the pediatrician will come to see your baby within twenty-four hours of delivery as well as once each day, until you go home. Choosing a doctor before delivery saves you the pressure of running around trying to do this after baby is born. If you have just delivered and are looking for a pediatrician right now, this chapter will also help you.

To get started, ask for names of pediatricians from friends, relatives, your obstetrician, nurse midwife, childbirth instructor, or people at work who have children. You can contact local medical societies or hospitals for information on which doctors have attended approved training programs and are board certified in pediatrics or family medicine. If it is possible, go with a friend to her baby's pediatric appointment to see what happens and become acquainted with the doctor's personality, attitudes, and style of care. Remember that what is important to your friend may or may not be important to you. When you have three or four names of physicians, call each one and talk over the phone, or better yet, arrange for a prenatal consultation. You may have to pay for such a meeting, but some physicians do not charge for a prenatal visit. If you belong to a prepaid health plan, there will be several physicians in the Pediatrics Department. Plan to visit at least one to become acquainted with this department. During your hospital stay you will probably come in contact with one or two other pediatricians as they take turns making rounds. Your final choice can be made after you go home. Fathers should plan on attending these prenatal consultations to get their questions answered and to realize that they may also be called upon to bring the baby to the doctor.

When advised to visit a pediatrician prenatally, many parents wonder, "What should I ask and take into consideration when making this choice?" What follows are some questions you can ask yourself and the doctor before you make your decision.

- Where is the office located in relation to your home? How easy is it to get there during the day, rush hour, and at night? Is there parking close by? Is the parking area well lit for night visits?
- Read about baby care issues before you go for the prenatal visit. Talk with other parents to find what they consider to be important issues. This helps you prepare your own set of questions.

- Ask the doctor if she has privileges at the hospital where you will be delivering. This means that even though she doesn't work at the hospital, she can examine and treat the baby there. If she does not have privileges there, who will see your baby? In a situation like this, it will usually be a staff pediatrician who will be assigned to care for your baby and stay in touch with your own doctor.

- Find out which hospital your child will be admitted into should he require hospitalization in the future. What are the special practices there in terms of visiting and rooming-in? Where would your child go in an emergency?

- What is the approximate size of the pediatrician's practice? How long do you have to wait for an appointment? How much time is set aside for each appointment? You should be seen within twenty minutes of your scheduled time.

- Who else is associated with the doctor? Does he have partners? Will you be seeing him or a partner for sick visits? Is there a nurse practitioner available for well-baby checks and daily parental concerns? Are there specific call-in times when the pediatrician or nurse practitioner is available for answering questions by phone?

- What are the arrangements for covering emergency calls and nights, weekends, and holidays? Does the doctor or nurse practitioner make house calls? Who covers when your doctor is on vacation?

- Find out what the costs are for office visits (well-child and sick-child), immunizations, consultations, emergency, or after hour visits. What fee adjustments can be made in relation to family income? What will your health insurance plan cover and what won't it cover? Ask this question if you belong to a prepaid health plan, too. Are there certain things that are not covered for which you will be charged? What is and is not covered during the hospital stay?

- What does the waiting room look like? Are there toys and books? How is it decorated? Does it look clean and well kept? Are there separate waiting areas for sick and well children? Are there laboratory facilities in the office for blood and urine tests, cultures, etc.? If not, where will you go for these services, as well as x rays and any other tests?

- How frequently will baby be seen during the first year? Is there a special payment plan for the first year of care? What is the immunization schedule?

- Ask the doctor's views on both bottle- and breastfeeding. When does she recommend starting solid foods? (Most babies do not need solids until they are between four and six months of age.) If you plan to breastfeed, ask what percentage of the practice consists of breastfed babies.

- What is the doctor's view on circumcision? It is now being debated, by those in the medical field, whether this procedure should be done only in special circumstances.

- How did you feel while talking to the doctor? Were you comfortable with how and what was being said? Did you notice any annoyance, boredom, or indifference to your questions and concerns? Were your questions answered fully, in language you could understand? Did the doctor seem to understand your fears and concerns? Were your needs as new parents addressed? If Dad went too, how did the physician relate to the prospective father? Did he direct his answers to both of you?

- Does the doctor seem concerned only with your baby's physical development and with treating disease, or is there also emphasis on mental development, behavior, and the parent-child relationship?

These are only suggested guidelines. You may have many other questions and concerns on which to base your final decision. Talk with each other about the information you have received. Take a list of questions with you, as you will not remember anything (except maybe your name) when you go for this visit. This paper will allow you to write down answers for review later. Your final selection of a pediatrician will be based on favorable responses to those topics that you feel are most important. Remember, in the end both you and your child go to the doctor!

Facts About Fever

New parents often become overly concerned when baby has a fever. Fever is a symptom that shows that the body is fighting disease or infection. If your baby has a fever of 102°F (39.9°C) or lower, most pediatricians recommend that you not try to lower the fever. You should call your doctor if your baby has a fever.

The most accurate way to determine if your baby has a fever is to take her temperature rectally. Of course, you must use a rectal thermometer to do this—don't use an oral thermometer!

To take your infant's temperature rectally, lie her on her side or abdomen. Be sure that you have placed your child in such way that there will be no sudden or forceful movement during the procedure. Lubricate the thermometer well with petroleum jelly and insert it ½ inch into the rectum. Hold it in place for four minutes, or until the mercury stops rising in the thermometer. It may be easier if two people are present during this procedure, as in Figure 7.5. You should know that the use of a rectal thermometer may stimulate bowel movement.

Many babies will fight against a rectal thermometer; for these babies, an axillary temperature can be taken. This can be done by placing the thermometer under baby's arm and holding her arm against her body. An axillary temperature will read about 1°F lower than a rectal temperature, but it will let you know if a fever is present.

You may also be able to determine whether baby has a fever by placing your lips on baby's forehead—the lips are much more sensitive to temperature than the hand.

You may wish to use one of the tape-like strips that are sold in many stores. These are placed on baby's forehead. Some types will tell you whether or not baby has a temperature, while others will give you the specific temperature. These may not be very accurate. There are also easy-to-read digital thermometers available.

The following chart shows the *normal* temperature for each method.

Normal Temperature	Method	Time
99.6°F (37.5°C)	Rectal	5 minutes
98.6°F (37.0°C)	Oral	3–5 minutes
97.6°F (35.5°C)	Axillary	10 minutes

INTERACTING WITH YOUR PEDIATRICIAN AFTER BABY IS BORN

In the Hospital

The next time you see your pediatrician (or maybe the first time) will be in the hospital within twenty-four hours of the birth. If you participate in an early discharge program, a staff pediatrician will check baby before you leave, and you will take baby to your own pediatrician in a few days. Most pediatricians make their morning rounds early. Ask your nurse to inform you when your pediatrician arrives so that you can meet her and watch the "newborn exam." This is a head-to-toe check to make sure that all systems are functioning properly. Your doctor will explain what she is checking for and show you all the special things that your newborn baby can do. You will enjoy watching this exam. It gives you a sense of who this little person is and allows you to ask questions to your heart's content.

One segment of this exam always fascinates parents—the check on the nervous system. Baby's nervous system is immature and characterized by a variety of reflexes. Baby shows uncoordinated movements, limited (but loud) means of communication, and little

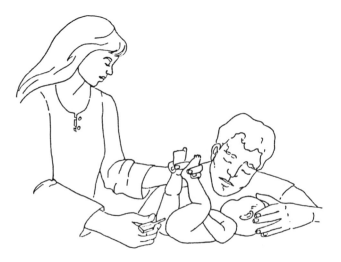

Figure 7.1.   Taking Baby's Temperature With a Rectal Thermometer

control over his bodily functions. These reflexes serve a variety of purposes. Some are protective (blinking, yawning, coughing, sneezing, drawing back from pain), some help in feeding (rooting, sucking, swallowing), and some encourage interaction with others (grasping).

A few of the most common reflexes that you will see the doctor check are listed and explained below.

Tonic Neck Reflex. (See Figure 7.2.) This is sometimes called the "fencer position." When baby is lying on his back, if his head is turned to one side, the arm and leg on that side will straighten, while the opposite arm and leg will flex. You may not see this reflex at first, but once it appears it will last until about four months of age.

Moro Reflex (startle reflex). (See Figure 7.3.) When baby is startled by a loud noise or is suddenly lowered in position, he will straighten his arms sideways and extend his fingers. His arms will slowly return to his chest like an embrace. His fingers will spread and form in a "C." This reflex is present at birth and disappears at between one and four months of age.

Grasp Reflex. (See Figure 7.4.) When baby's palm is stimulated with a finger or object he will grasp and hold it firmly enough to be lifted momentarily from a flat surface. This reflex lessens when the baby is about five months old.

Rooting Reflex. (See Figure 1.2.) When the side of the baby's mouth or cheek is touched, he will turn toward that side and open his mouth. This disappears by seven months of age. This reflex is difficult to elicit after a feeding.

Sucking Reflex. When an object is placed in baby's mouth, he begins sucking on it. This reflex disappears at around twelve months of age.

Stepping Reflex. (See Figure 7.5.) When baby is held upright with one foot touching a flat surface, he will put one foot in front of the other and "walk." This reflex disappears in one or two months.

Before you leave the hospital, your pediatrician or nurse practitioner will talk to you about the next few weeks at home. She will tell you when she next wants to see the baby. This next visit is usually on the tenth to fourteenth day after birth and will include a weight check if baby is breastfed. Some bottle-fed babies may have this visit at two to four weeks of age. These times vary, so check with your doctor.

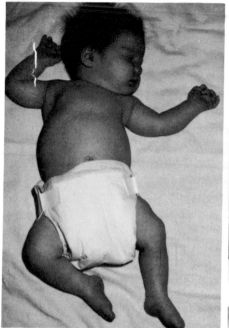

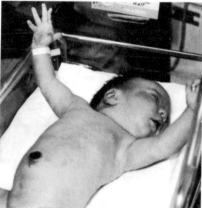

◀ **Figure 7.2.**
The Tonic Neck Reflex

▼ **Figure 7.3.**
The Moro Reflex

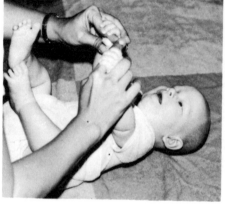

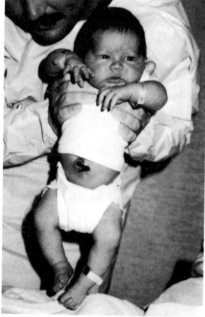

Figure 7.4. ▲
The Grasp Reflex

Figure 7.5. ➤
The Stepping Reflex

Your pediatrician or maternity nurse will probably also explain other nursery procedures such as the vitamin K injection. Babies are routinely given an injection of vitamin K (and you thought vitamins only went to E!) on the day of their birth. Vitamin K is one of many factors necessary for the blood to clot. Because babies lack vitamin K for the first few days after birth, they are given some to tide them over until their body starts making it.

Another test that will be done on your baby is the PKU Test. **Phenylketonuria** (PKU) is an uncommon inborn error of metabolism. The incidence of this disorder is about one for every 10,000 to 20,000 births. A baby with PKU lacks a certain liver enzyme that breaks down the amino acid called **phenylalanine**. Amino acids are the building blocks of protein. Phenylalanine is an essential amino acid used by the body for growth. A baby with PKU cannot break down this amino acid, so it accumulates in the blood and eventually spills into the urine. Excesssive amounts of phenylalanine in the tissues can lead to progressive mental retardation.

Testing for PKU is mandatory in many states. If it is not required in your state, check with your pediatrician to see how this testing will be handled. In the nursery, a small amount of baby's blood is taken from his heel and sent to a lab for testing. A second test may be done four to six weeks later to determine the results after milk feedings have been well established.

Some parents will do a diaper test for PKU. You will be given a specially prepared test paper either by the hospital or your doctor. At about six weeks of age you will take a freshly wet diaper and press the prepared test paper against the wet area of the diaper. You will follow the directions for reporting the results. If PKU is identified, special diets and formula can be given to limit the intake of phenylalanine. Many babies can also continue to breast-feed, if watched carefully.

At the Doctor's Office

Your first visit to the pediatrician or nurse practitioner will probably be a very exciting one for you for several reasons.

- You will want to see how baby is doing and be assured that he is healthy and gaining weight.
- You will have the opportunity to ask, in an offhand manner,

all the questions that you were afraid to call about for fear of sounding like a crazed new parent!

- You will be able to get out of the bathrobe you have been living in for the past two weeks!

This visit will be around two weeks (sometimes earlier) for a weight check and general examination of baby. Take a list of questions with you. The pediatrician or nurse practitioner will weigh baby, and measure his length and head circumference to make sure his head and brain are growing properly. Baby's eyes will be checked, as will his heart and lungs. His abdomen and hips will be checked for dislocation and he will get the once-over all the way to his toes. Immunizations will be discussed and will generally start in the second month.

One more hint. Some babies are quiet and relaxed for this visit. Other babies, however, may scream their heads off at this intrusion into their lives. Don't go crazy if your baby cries the entire time you are in the exam room. The fastest way to calm baby is to allow him to suck on your finger or on a pacifier while being gently rocked. Don't bounce, jiggle, or yell at baby—he can't help it! Ask if most of the exam can be conducted while you hold baby on your lap. This is only the beginning—wait until he needs stitches!

Immunization

Infants are immunized against polio, diphtheria, pertussis (whooping cough), tetanus, measles, mumps, rubella (German measles), and at two years of age a particular type of influenza. The polio immunization is given orally and the rest are injections. A TB (tuberculosis) test is usually performed at twelve months. Occasionally, a baby has a bad reaction to the pertussis (whooping cough) part of the DPT shot. Ask your nurse practitioner or pediatrician what to look for, and don't hesitate to call him if your baby exhibits any of the symptoms he describes.

The chart below is a typical schedule of visits and immunizations, although some pediatricians and family practitioners routinely schedule more frequent visits, especially if it is your first baby. Lead screening can also be done should you or your physician or nurse practitioner feel that it is necessary.

Table 7.1   Immunization Chart

Age	Immunization
2 weeks	
2 months	DPT (diphtheria, pertussis, and tetanus) and polio
4 months	DPT and polio
6 months	DPT
9 months	
12 months	Tuberculine Test
15 months	MMR (measles, mumps, rubella)
	Baby must be a full 15 months for the immunization
18 months	DPT and polio
2 years	HIB (influenza shot)

Chapter Eight

Your Physical Recovery From Childbirth

It took your body nine months of gradual and specialized change to grow your baby. Now it is asked to respond rapidly to not being pregnant.

Many of the changes that occur after birth are automatic (shrinking of the uterus, eliminating excess fluid) while others take some effort on your part (toning of the abdominal and pelvic floor muscles). Many mothers are in a great hurry to get things back to the way they used to be. Be aware, however, that your body may not return to exactly how it looked before you were pregnant. At five days postpartum you are not going to look like those skinny models on the covers of fashion magazines, and you're not supposed to! Be patient. Try to ignore friends and family who keep staring at your sagging belly. We always wonder what it is they expect to see! This section will discuss some of the physical changes you will experience during the postpartum period.

INVOLUTION OF THE UTERUS

Following the expulsion or delivery of the placenta (also called afterbirth), the uterus contracts to the size of a large grapefruit. Each day thereafter the uterus gets smaller and descends further down into the pelvis until, after two weeks, you cannot feel it anymore when you press on the abdomen. This shrinking process is called **involution**. If you are breastfeeding, this process may occur more quickly, as the same hormone that causes milk to be delivered to the baby also causes the uterus to contract.

This is a safeguard to prevent you from losing too much blood from the placental site.

Many mothers, especially if they are breastfeeding, are aware of what are called "after pains." These are contractions that occur when you put baby to breast the first few days after delivery. Mothers who have had their second or subsequent baby are often more aware of these. When the baby nurses, the uterus must work to contract, causing cramping and some pain. These pains will gradually stop after a few days. If they are very painful, try using your breathing and relaxation techniques.

Your cervix, which was dilated (opened) to ten centimeters (four inches), during delivery, is now soft and spongy, but will firm up and close by the end of seven days.

VAGINA

The vagina, which was stretched during the baby's passage, will gradually reduce in size but will not be the same as before the birth. Slackness or low tone of the muscles surrounding the vaginal opening can be taken care of by pelvic floor muscle exercises (called **Kegel exercises**). You will slowly contract and relax the muscles that control the start and stop of urination. These exercises are done in sets of five, ten times per day. This is an important part of your recovery, as failure to tighten up these very stretched muscles can sometimes lead to urinary incontinence (leaking of urine when pressure or stress is put on these muscles such as when you cough, laugh, or sneeze), and reduction of the pleasurable sensations felt during intercourse.

The pelvic floor muscles support the pelvic organs. If they are allowed to remain slack, then the bladder, uterus, and rectum have lost some of their support. This can sometimes lead to a prolapse of one of these organs, which means that the organ has moved down and out of place. These exercises are important whether or not you have had an episiotomy.

EPISIOTOMY

An **episiotomy** is a surgical cut that enlarges the vaginal opening during childbirth. This procedure has become controversial, since some doctors do it routinely and others only if really necessary. If you had an episiotomy, the perineum will still be somewhat tender, sore, and swollen, and may be bruised from the delivery. Kegel exercises, sitz baths, and hot, wet compresses usually help increase the circulation to that area, and promote healing. Ice packs can be applied for the first twenty-four hours to decrease swelling. If you had an episiotomy, the stitches will dissolve over a week or so. They are not removed at a doctor's office. Use the treatments described above for comfort. You will be shown how to care for your perineum in the hospital. You may also notice that the labia become flabby after childbearing. This is normal.

LOCHIA

Lochia is a bloody discharge from the uterus that continues for about two to four weeks following childbirth. Lochia is composed of blood from where the placenta was attached and pieces of the lining of the uterus that is sloughed off. Over the first three or four days, the lochia is bright red and may contain small clots. It gradually changes in color and composition so that over the next five to ten days it becomes pinker and less in quantity. After that it turns a yellowish-white and finally stops. Report excessive clotting or large clots to your doctor, nurse practitioner, or nurse midwife. You will wear sanitary napkins, not tampons, during this time to decrease the chance of an infection occurring through the open cervix. The general pattern described above also occurs in mothers who have had a Cesarean delivery, although lochia tends to occur in lesser amounts and for a shorter period of time. Mothers have told us that this must make up for nine months of having no periods!

If you notice that the amount of lochia increases or the color turns back to a bright red, then you are probably overexerting yourself. Trying to be supermom and telling yourself that the baby won't change your life is pointless. Overdoing it by entertaining, lifting, and tearing up and down the stairs with laundry slows the process of involution and healing. This is a time to regroup and take care of yourself. Otherwise, you'll end up with a massive case of burnout and fatigue before you've been a parent a month!

Call your health care provider if any of the following situations occur.

- There is a sudden or large amount of bright red blood from the vagina after the lochia has decreased and changed in color.
- You are faint, dizzy, or so exhausted that you cannot function.
- The lochia has a foul odor or changes to other than what has been described above.
- Large clots or small clots with a heavy flow occur.
- You are soaking more than one pad an hour.

Lochia may also:
- Stop for a few days and start up again.
- Gush when you first get up from bed in the morning.
- Spurt when you breastfeed.
- Occur in increased amounts after urination.
- Occur in increased amounts with women having their second or subsequent baby.
- Decrease when you are lying down.

ABDOMEN

Many women think that they will be able to pour themselves into size three designer jeans a couple of hours after delivery. Wrong! The abdominal wall has been stretched by the pregnancy and it will take a couple of months to stop looking like you are still five months pregnant! This may sound discouraging, but the news is not all bad. If you have exercised and used these muscles during pregnancy, they tend to regain their tone much faster with proper diet, rest, and exercise. This may take longer with mothers of twins, mothers who have had one or more babies, or women who had poor tone to begin with. You may not fit into your regular clothes for a while. Consider wearing slacks with elastic waists and roomy sweaters or blouses.

Today, most women will start some sort of exercise program when their health care provider gives the go-ahead. The earliest exercises are usually the ones you learned in your childbirth classes or from handouts you receive with exercise instructions.

Do not do any exercises that cause pain, increase lochia, or tire you out.

There are many organized exercise programs for both prenatal and postpartum women. The YWCA, women's centers, HMO's (health maintenance organizations), childbirth education groups, hospitals, and health clubs are a few ideas. Avoid following exercise videotapes that may be too vigorous or have exercises that may cause injury. If you have particular questions, special needs, or wish to have an exercise program developed just for you, try consulting a physical therapist, or look for exercise classes led by a physical therapist.

You may notice stretch marks on the outside of your abdomen. These occur as a result of the stretching and rupture of the elastic fibers in your skin. They are reddish-purple after delivery and will gradually fade in time to appear as white or silver streaks. They may also be seen on the breasts, thighs, and buttocks. No amount of cocoa butter, creams, lotions, or "goops" can prevent this prenatally or fix it postpartum. Don't spend outrageous amounts of money on heavily advertised products that, at best, will only moisturize your skin.

HUNGER AND NUTRITION

You may be very hungry after your baby is born and will be given food and fluid then, as well as three meals a day in the hospital. Good nutrition is an important part of your physical recovery from pregnancy and childbirth. After you get home you may find that you have a ravenous appetite, or you may have little interest in food, especially if you have to fix the food yourself. You must continue to eat a well-balanced diet, just as you did in pregnancy. Choose foods high in iron and protein for iron replacement and tissue healing.

If you are breastfeeding you also need some good sources of calcium. However, you don't have to drink milk to make milk. Many adults do not care for or cannot tolerate milk. Pick up calcium from green vegetables, cheese, yogurt, cottage cheese, or salmon. There are no food restrictions for breastfeeding mothers. Eat foods from the four basic food groups: milk and dairy, meat and fish, fruit and vegetables, and bread and grains.

You do not give your baby gas from the foods you consume. If you like baked beans, broccoli, and brussel sprouts, then eat them. You'll be the one in the bathroom! Some strong seasonings will occcasionally flavor your milk, but unless you have a baby with a real discriminating palate, this will not be a problem. If your baby screams for hours after you have eaten pepperoni, garlic, onions, or whatever, and this happens every time, then don't eat them! Most of the mothers in the world eat spices with no problems. Placing lists of restrictions on food for nursing mothers is useless. It causes you to eliminate healthy items from your diet for no real reason.

Digestive upsets sometimes occur in susceptible nursing babies when large quantities of cow's milk are consumed by Mom. Cow's milk protein is the major allergen in childhood. If you notice that your baby suffers from long periods of inconsolable crying, eczema-like rashes, or a runny nose, try eliminating milk from your diet for a few weeks.

Some breastfeeding mothers need to increase their calorie intake by about 500 calories (1,000 with twins) or adjust their calories so that they are slowly losing weight and are not fatigued to the point of not being able to function. The fluid requirement for a nursing mother is about simply drinking to thirst. Do not overdo the fluids—too much is not good either. Water, juices, and soups are fine.

Limit your intake of caffeine-containing beverages to about one serving per day. Caffeine is a drug that babies have difficulty ridding from their systems. It therefore can accumulate and cause jittery, fussy, and awake babies. Keep in mind that caffeine is found not only in coffee and tea but also in many soft drinks.

Alcohol is another drug that nursing mothers ask about. Some mothers are given the old advice about drinking a glass of beer a day to increase their energy or to help them relax before a feeding. This is not necessary, as there are no nutritional elements in beer that cannot be found elsewhere. Drinking a glass of beer each time you nurse, ten or twelve times in twenty-four hours, is absurd and will only interfere with your parenting abilities and the letting down of milk. Not to mention what that level of alcohol would do to the baby! *Moderation* is the key. A glass of beer or wine with dinner is not a problem. Large quantities of alcohol are not desirable. Small amounts can increase prolactin levels, but this does not mean that larger amounts increase milk supply.

"But what about chocolate? I love chocolate!" Chocolate contains a substance that is chemically similar to caffeine. So here again, moderation is the key. A chocolate bar is fine—but not the whole chocolate cake or pound of choice goodies!

If you are bottle feeding your baby, good nutrition is still important for your recovery. A well-balanced diet in amounts that will allow you to lose weight gradually is desirable. Crash, fad, or variety-restricted diets are not a good idea. They rob you of your energy and often do not provide enough nutrients for repair of tissues and replacement of iron. A breastfeeding mother's body will take two to three hundred calories per day from fat stores laid down during pregnancy and put them into the milk and making of milk. This will not happen to mothers who bottle feed, but there is no reason why they will not gradually lose weight too.

Weight loss and getting one's figure back are high priorities for many women in our thin-thinking culture. Staying away from junk food and setting reasonable weight loss goals are appropriate. Avoid spas and health clubs that advise strict calorie limits or do not have special postpartum exercise programs.

Some mothers find that they are not very hungry and have little desire to fix nutritious meals for themselves. One way to assure that the food is prepared is to have someone help you out the first few weeks you are home. Friends who wish to help can be asked to prepare casseroles, stews, soups, or other foods that can be stored or frozen and used for two meals. Some mothers will freeze several meals before the baby is born.

Snacking is another easy way to obtain needed food, especially if you do not have a large appetite. Snacks that help with daily food requirements include carrots, yogurt, nuts, cheese, peanut butter and crackers, dried fruits, hard boiled eggs, oranges, apples, bananas, green peppers, etc. Avoid candy, cookies, donuts, cakes, and other calorie-rich but nutritionally poor foods. Have a bowl of fresh fruit sitting out in your kitchen and raw vegetables in a bowl in your refrigerator. Breastfeeding mothers, and some bottle feeding mothers, are advised to continue taking their prenatal vitamins for a few months after delivery. Remember that you must take care of yourself before you can take care of others.

If you experienced a Cesarean delivery, you will not be fed immediately in the recovery room. Usually it takes a couple of days before your intestines are ready to move things along. You will start out on clear liquids in the hospital, then soft foods, and finally solid foods as soon as you are ready. When you get home, the above recommendations still hold. A balanced diet with protein at each meal helps you recover from both child-birth and surgery.

Sometimes gas can be an early problem. Avoid carbonated beverages and gas-producing foods. Early frequent movement in bed and walking in the hospital will help.

If you have particular questions or problems or require spe-cialized diet planning, consult a nutritionist who can tailor meal-planning to your needs.

ELIMINATION

Urination

You may have found it somewhat difficult to urinate right after you gave birth. If you had regional anesthesia it is hard to pee when you are not aware that your bladder is full. Even if you had no anesthesia, swelling and bruising around the urinary opening may decrease the usual sensitivity to when it is time to go. Starting the Kegel (pelvic floor muscles) exercises immedi-ately may help stimulate urination. Slow chest breathing, relaxa-tion techniques, standing up, or perineal care with warm water will also help.

If you have not urinated within a certain number of hours after delivery (this varies from place to place) you will be cathe-terized. This is because an overfull bladder increases the chance of a urinary tract infection and may displace the uterus, which interferes with its ability to contract, thereby allowing a large blood loss. This is not a common event but it sometimes hap-pens. A hollow tube is passed into the bladder to drain it. This is more commonly done to mothers who have had regional anes-thesia such as caudal, epidural, and spinal blocks. All mothers who have had a Cesarean delivery have been catheterized.

Being catheterized increases the risk of a urinary tract infection. Be on the lookout for its symptoms, which include frequent and painful urination, a burning sensation while urinating, chills, fever, back pains, and urinating very small amounts very frequently. If you have questions, call your health care provider.

Bowels

Did you ever think that you would have to read about this!

The bowels tend to be sluggish after delivery. This is usually caused by decreased hormonal levels, decreased muscle tone in the intestines, and decreased pressure in the abdomen. The questionable and outmoded practice of administering an enema in early labor contributes to this problem, as does going for a long period of time without food. Sometimes constipation can result, especially if a mother delays having a bowel movement because of pain from hemorrhoids, or fears that she will damage the perineum or tear stitches.

You may not have a bowel movement until the second or third day following delivery. Some mothers experience diarrhea right before they go into labor. So where is the body supposed to gather enough waste materials in a short hospital stay to have a bowel movement before going home? Some health care providers insist that women move their bowels before being discharged from the hospital, and prescribe medication to insure that this happens. Check this one out with your own care giver.

Some ways to help stimulate bowel function are to drink plenty of fluids, eat cooked or fresh fruit, bran muffins, or bran cereal, or sprinkle 100 percent bran into foods. Prunes or prune juice helps, as do whole-grain breads and leafy vegetables. If none of this seems to help, you can try a product that produces bulk in the intestines. Stool softeners can be used that soften the bowel movement so that you won't be afraid of the pain. Do not take laxatives. This practice gets your body into the bad habit of relying on them for each bowel movement.

Hemorrhoids (We can hear you groaning!)

Oh, yes—there is this too! You may have been aware of hemorrhoids during your pregnancy, and it is certainly common to
experience them after having a baby. Hemorrhoids are enlarged
blood vessels that protrude out of the anal opening. They result
from the pressure put on them during a pregnancy and from
the pushing during the second stage of labor. Hemorrhoids
resemble little finger-like projections of flesh. They are the lit-
eral pain in the rear! They make it difficult to sit or get comfortable and can be very painful, and sometimes even bleed. Hemorrhoids usually clear up in ten to fourteen days following
delivery. In the meantime, you can try any or all of the
following.

- A sitz bath for your entire bottom.
- Contracting the anal muscles several times after pushing the
  hemorrhoids back into the anal opening.
- Applying any one of a number of ointments that contain an
  anesthetic or special ingredients for hemorrhoids. (Check
  with your health care provider.)
- Applying gauze pads soaked in medication or witch hazel.
- Cold packs for twenty-four hours following delivery.

WEIGHT CHANGES IN THE IMMEDIATE
POSTPARTUM PERIOD

You will lose about ten pounds or so immediately after delivery.
This represents the weight of the baby, placenta, and amniotic
fluid. You will lose another three pounds or so during the next
week as your body rids itself of extra fluid. Your body does this
by increasing the amount of urine output, especially during the
first twelve to twenty-four hours. Two to three quarts of fluid will
be eliminated with a normal pregnancy, and more if you have
experienced pre-eclampsia or eclampsia (toxemia), high blood
pressure, or diabetes.

You will notice that excess fluid and waste products are also
eliminated through the skin by an increased amount of perspi-
ration. Sweating episodes frequently occur at night, and you
may awaken drenched in sweat. Towels and an extra nightgown

may be needed at these times. A daily shower will help keep you refreshed. This condition doesn't last long!

SKIN CHANGES AND PIGMENTATION

You may have have noticed, during your pregnancy, what are called "spiders." These are thin, red, branching lines that appear on various parts of your body. "Spiders" are dilated (distended) capillaries close to the surface of the skin. They tend to fade and may regress within a couple of months following delivery.

During pregnancy you may have also seen increased pigmentation or a darker coloring on certain areas of your body, especially the areas that already have darker skin—the genitals, areolae, nipples, and around the navel. Some women develop freckles or dark, mask-like coloring on the face and around the eyes. The *linea nigra* is a dark line from the navel to the pubic hair that will lighten in time, as will the areas on your face.

RETURN OF MENSTRUATION

When you resume your monthly periods is variable. If you are not breastfeeding, your first period may occur six to eight weeks after delivery. If you are breastfeeding, your period may not return for many months. If you totally nurse your baby with no skipped feedings, bottles, solid foods, or long stretches of time when the breasts do not receive stimulation, then ovulation is suppressed. However, it is possible to resume your periods anytime when you are nursing, especially when the number or frequency of feedings is reduced. Your normal cycle may become a little irregular for a while, with skipped or shortened periods. Some women find that their cycles become very regular if they were not before. If baby starts to increase the number of feedings again because of a growth spurt, teething, or illness, then ovulation may once again stop for a month or two.

Having your period while nursing a baby does not affect the quality or quantity of milk. Nor is there any proof that it changes the breastfeeding relationship.

It is quite possible to become pregnant soon after you give birth, whether or not you are breastfeeding. Breastfeeding is not a contraceptive. It usually spaces children about two years apart if contraceptive measures are not used.

RECOVERY FROM A CESAREAN DELIVERY

Most of what we have been discussing in this chapter so far applies if you are anticipating or have experienced either a Cesarean delivery or a vaginal delivery. There are, however, a few other things to discuss that will be of help during your recovery from Cesarean childbirth.

Initial Feedings

Some Cesarean births are scheduled in advance, or mothers know that they will have a Cesarean when they begin labor. These circumstances arise from personal choice or from a situation that makes vaginal delivery undesirable, dangerous, or impossible. For many other mothers, Cesarean delivery is a surprise—and a sometimes disappointing one. In a situation like this, some women feel cheated out of a special experience. They may feel guilty and angry, and that things are completely out of their control. In addition, pain, isolation, loneliness, and immobility slow down the process of getting the new family off to a good start. All of these feelings are normal. Usually, as you start to feel physically better and get moving, your inner feelings lift too.

Most women need to talk about their labor and delivery to help validate that what happened was right and to make sure that they have all the details. This allows the experience to become part of who they are. This process is very important to a woman who had an operative delivery. Ask if you can talk to the labor and delivery nurse who took care of you. She can help review what happened and put things in perspective. Talk to your baby's father or whomever was your support person. Their views and observations are helpful, too. If you feel that you need more help, ask to speak to a nurse who is a mental health clinical specialist. She will help you sort out all those conflicting emotions.

Some mothers find that they are just relieved that the baby is healthy, and that holding and feeding the baby help with the disappointment. Your view of a Cesarean delivery may be that it is another of life's events to be experienced (or endured) with optimism and patience.

Tips for in the Hospital

Getting Out of Bed

While you are in the hospital you should move around as soon as you can. Start by dangling your legs off the side of the bed, and then begin to walk as soon as you are able.

You should ask for assistance the first few times that you get up. You may feel weak and dizzy, and we don't want new mothers to fall down! Abdominal tightening exercises and deep breathing can be done in your bed before you get up.

Request an electrically controlled bed. If you don't have one, ask someone to crank up the bed before you get out. Rather than trying to do a situp when you first want to get out of bed, raise the back of the bed all the way up first, then get out. When you first get up, it may feel as though your incision is going to split open. It won't, because it is stitched together on the inside and either stitched, clamped, or stapled on the outside. But talk is cheap! Most women feel better when they splint the incision while getting up or turning in bed. Make a splint with the fingers of both hands laced together and placed over the incision. (See Figure 8.1.) This helps you feel better (both physically

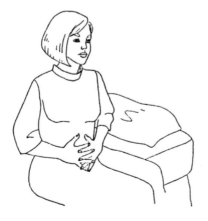

Figure 8.1.   Splinting the Cesarean Incision

and mentally) when you move. Remember to stand up straight and not to stoop when you walk.

Feeding Your Baby

We suggest that you keep your baby in bed with you so that you don't have to reach or lift at feeding time. If you are breastfeeding, use the football hold to keep the weight of the baby off your incision. (See Figure 2.4.) Some mothers with a low incision find that a pillow on the lap takes most of the baby's weight, allowing more of a variety of nursing positions to be used.

A Cesarean delivery does not change any of the mechanisms of breastfeeding. Sometimes babies are separated from a Cesarean-delivered mother because people mistakenly think that she can't take care of the baby or that she doesn't want the baby until she feels better. This is rarely true. Sometimes maternal complications occur, but more often mothers are just tired and need a little extra help the first few days. Make your feelings known.

Get Some Rest!

Rest as much as possible. Limit visitors and telephone calls. Put a "Do Not Disturb" sign on your door during visiting hours if the whole neighborhood and all your relatives decide that you need company in the hospital—you don't. If they want to help, tell them to clean your house, stock your refrigerator and freezer, and run any last-minute errands.

The following are some other suggestions that you may find helpful while you are in the hospital.

- Do not compare your progress of recovery with other Cesarean mothers or mothers who vaginally delivered. You will recover at your own rate and in your own way.
- Use pain medication as needed. Small amounts taken for a couple of days will not harm the baby if you are breastfeeding.
- Get up and shower as soon as your doctor says you can. This will make you feel much better. The incision will be covered by a big bandage that is usually removed in a couple of days, and you can shower while wearing the bandage.

Most skin incisions are made across the pubic hair line (bikini, smile, transverse, pfannensteil). Sometimes a midline or classical incision is made from below the navel to the pubic hair line when circumstances do not allow the lower incision. Your nurse and physician will check the incision daily to make sure it is healing properly and not showing signs of infection.

- Request that a student nurse be assigned to you. She will usually be of great help during your first few days in the hospital as she may have more time to spend with you.

Tips for the First Weeks Home After Cesarean Delivery

- *Get help!* Most women hate to be dependent on others for help, but after childbirth and surgery you deserve and need it.
- Your physician may or may not have outlined restrictions on your activities. Some doctors will give you a list of do's and don'ts, while others feel that common sense and your own body will tell you how much you can do.
- Plan on doing nothing for two weeks except resting, eating, and feeding baby. Relatives and friends can help as long as they don't create more problems than they solve and don't make you a nervous wreck. Your job is not to entertain people. Limit friends to a five-minute visit with you. Wear a bathrobe so they won't overstay! If they really want to help, tell them to bring dinner on disposable dishes.
- Report any of the following to your nurse practitioner or physician:

  —Lochia changes, as described earlier in this chapter.
  —Pain or burning with urination, as already mentioned.
  —Incision pain, discharge, foul odor, or change in color (itching is normal).

- Fever.
- Any other pains for which you cannot account.

Many women worry that because they had a Cesarean delivery they will always have to have Cesarean deliveries. This is no longer true. For many women, vaginal delivery is possible with the next baby, depending on what the reason was for the first

Cesarean. If it is a non-repeating condition and if the mother meets the criteria set for a vaginal birth after a Cesarean (VBAC), then she is usually encouraged to attempt a vaginal delivery.

Although a Cesarean delivery places extra stress on the family, it is still the birth of a baby. With love, patience, communication, and support, the initial difficulties and frustrations will give way to a thriving family with a cherished new member.

This chapter has addressed the common physical changes that occur following childbirth. But there are also emotional adjustments to make. The next four chapters will look at the emotional side of new parenthood and the roles and relationships surrounding this event.

Chapter Nine

Postpartum Emotional Adjustments

Do you *feel* like a mother or a father? Just what should being a parent feel like? It is not uncommon, as you gaze at your sleeping newborn, to wonder when his parents will arrive, because you do not feel as though you are old enough to be a parent! Have faith—this transition into parenthood does not occur overnight. It takes time to become a psychological mother or father.

Remember the first job you had when you completed your schooling? Did you feel confident and secure on your first day? Or did you feel anxious, confused, or clumsy? Did you spend a lot of time worrying about how you would perform, or if people would like you? Well, parenting is a job, too. It is not an instinctive, natural process that occurs just because you have biologically given birth. It is a learned role, one that combines behavior, intuition, consistent information, and lots of honesty, as well as humor. Parenthood is a stage of life that is filled with many emotions.

Because of the complexity of this role development, you should relax your expectations of yourself and your child. You will never be the "perfect parent," and you will never have the "perfect child."

Now, with that out of the way, let's talk about the feelings and emotions that will accompany this new phase in your life—living with your new baby.

You are now home with your new baby. Was it an easy ride from the hospital, or did it take twice as long as it should have because you had to go down all the back roads to avoid the traffic? It is not uncommon for a new mother to arrive at home and find about twenty people waiting for her at the front door! They say, "We didn't want to see you in the hospital—we thought you might be tired!" Little do they know that, at this point, you feel as though you have just run a marathon.

What about these visitors? What should you do? You will probably want to ask them all to leave. But you will not have the emotional energy to do that, so you will all sit around while they o-o-o-h and a-a-h over your baby. They probably all brought presents for the baby, and after about an hour you may begin to wonder if you were there for the birth! You will begin to feel a bit dethroned. This is very normal. Remember, when you were pregnant, you were the center of attention. Many people were concerned with how you felt and if you were comfortable. With the birth of the baby, it is not uncommon to feel as though you have faded into the background. It is important to acknowledge the emotion and not feel bad about your feelings. In your mind you may be thinking, "Now this is silly. I should be happy that everyone is enjoying my baby. Why do I feel as though I want to sit down and cry?"

Have you ever heard of the "baby blues"? Mood swings, confusion, fatigue, irritability, and anxiety are common symptoms of this period. Baby blues can occur in about 50 to 80 percent of women who give birth. It is a time when your hormones have taken a plunge, and you feel a kind of letdown. The blues generally peak at the fifth day after the birth and subside about two weeks after the birth. At this time you feel that if anyone looks at you funny, you will cry. Are you going crazy, you may wonder? No, you are not. Let's talk about what may be going on.

FANTASY VS. REALITY

During pregnancy, we all have dreams and fantasies about what we will be like as mothers. You may have attended classes that prepared you for childbirth and learned how to work with your body during the experience of labor and delivery. It was great— you enjoyed lying on the floor with pillows and relaxing during the breathing exercises. It was all perfect on the theory level. But what happened when reality struck? Did you feel in complete control during the contractions, or did you pray for some magical thing to happen to make it all go away? Had you planned on avoiding Cesarean delivery, anesthesia, and episiot- omy? These dreams and fantasies were great on the abstract level, but when you were really experiencing labor, it was hard work. What happened?

Many women will begin to mentally "work through" their birth experience on about the third day after the birth. That is when they are beginning to have enough energy to even think about it. It is in this period of "working through" that women begin to analyze their performance and become critics. They now look back on the birth and forget what they were feeling at the time. It is at this time that many woman will describe going through a period of mourning their "perfect birth." With this mourning they may feel sad, confused, and full of wonder about why they did not "do it right."

It is important for you to talk with your partner, physician, midwife, or nurse about what you are feeling. See if you can fill in the "missing pieces" of the birth. You were very involved, on both a physical and emotional level, with the job at hand— delivering your baby—so you will need the feedback and input of those who were in attendance to complete the picture. Many women may feel as though they did not "bond" at birth: "After I saw that she was all right, all I wanted to do was go to sleep. I was exhausted and shaking...then when I woke up, I felt bad! I didn't bond at birth!"

It is important to consider from the beginning that if you don't take care of yourself, you will not have the energy to care for your baby. You have plenty of time to grow in attachment with your baby...relax and be careful about becoming your own worst critic. You did the best you could, and that is all you will ever do.

So what about these feelings? If you want to cry, then cry. Crying real hard is a wonderful way to relieve anxiety and to promote relaxation. Think of the times in your life when you have sobbed. Afterwards, didn't you feel better? Didn't you sink into a deep sleep? Well, that is what you need now.

It is important to share your feelings with someone you trust. How about your husband? He may have similar feelings. What a way to share. Wrap your arms around each other and cry. Put the birth into perspective so that you can begin to direct your energies toward learning to live with this baby.

POSTPARTUM DEPRESSIVE SYNDROME

If you should find that you are not feeling emotionally intact for longer than two weeks, and that you are wondering why you feel so sad and, at times, immobilized, then it is time to seek additional support. **Postpartum depressive syndrome** (also known as **maternal depressive syndrome**) occurs in about 10–20 percent of woman who give birth. It is a syndrome that is finally beginning to be recognized in our society. It can begin after about three weeks, or may be delayed four to five months postpartum. It is accompanied by feelings of anxiety, panic, irritability, phobias, and/or sadness. Many women will feel a loss of identity, as though they don't know who they are. There are no sure causes of this syndrome—it may have a biochemical link. It may also be related to adapting to the role of motherhood. In today's society, woman are expected to "get it all together" after the birth. There are limited role models and few extended families in our society today. Many women will go home from the hospital to an empty house or apartment during the day, while their husband-/boyfriend is at work. If you worked full time prior to the birth, you may not have developed a new network of friends who are also mothers. You have no idea what feelings are normal, and you may isolate yourself even further because you think you should be feeling so happy, yet you feel so sad. You have received little, if any, preparation for *living* with the baby, but feel as though you were saturated with information about how to *have* the baby.

If you are experiencing this syndrome, it is important that you seek professional help. Maternal depressive syndrome can be treated with psychotherapy and/or medication. It is very helpful to become involved in a mother's support group so that you will know that you are not alone. These support groups also provide wonderful sharing times and opportunities for relationship development.

Because this syndrome is beginning to be recognized, it is imperative that you seek help from a professional person who is up-to-date on the treatment and management of postpartum depression (psychiatrist, psychologist, psychiatric clinical nurse specialist, and/or licensed social worker). With the correct treatment and intervention, you will recover and grow from the experience.

There is a more severe postpartum emotional reaction called postpartum psychosis. This occurs in about 1–2 percent of childbearing women. Mothers who have this disorder lose contact with reality, may experience suicidal or homicidal urges, and require immediate hospitalization. This disorder is rare, but you should be aware of it.

As you can see, postpartum is a time of psychological vulnerability. Therefore, it is important that you care for yourself after the birth. You are a very important person.

Suggestions for Taking Care of Yourself and Your New Emotions

- Your sleep/rest needs are important.... if you don't enjoy taking naps, then arrange to have "quiet time" at least once during the day when you do something for *you*. Some examples would be:

  —Sit in a comfortable chair, turn on some soft, relaxing music, and do relaxation breathing. All too often, the skills that you may have learned in the Preparation for Childbirth classes are forgotten after the birth. In many ways these skills are even more important in the post-birth phase.

  Some women have found that using a stress reduction audiotape is helpful because they can follow the voice on the tape and enter a relaxed state at a quicker pace. This all depends on your own skill level. Be aware that the voice on the tape is important. Make sure it is relaxing to you!

  —Take time to read the morning paper and have a cup of coffee or tea (decaffeinated may be the better choice). This is a luxury that you may have been dreaming of but have not fit into your day. The housework will get done. Many household tasks can be accomplished while the baby sits in an infant seat on the floor during a wakeful period and watches you!

- Simplify your life:
  —Paper plates and cups will decrease the amount of dishes staring at you in the sink. They are available all year long, and why use china for toast or a sandwich?
  —"Declutter" your house or apartment so that there are not a lot of "things" sitting around. It is especially important to have one neat room that you enjoy being in where you can feed the baby or just sit and relax. Very often women have shared that they felt that if their house was clean, they were more in control. But if that means that you are spending four hours a day doing housework, when do you rest? Remember, the housework will be there no matter how old your child, but that this phase of personal, physical, and emotional recovery is necessary *now.*
  —Buy a telephone answering machine. This is a wonderful way for you to control the interruptions in your day and allow yourself to rest and recover. You can hear who is calling and decide if you want to talk. If it is a person you do not feel like talking to or about business that you do not feel like discussing now, then let the machine take the message! The telephone is a major source of interruptions and it is also a piece of equipment that, at times, tries to rule your life. *You have control over it!*

- Your home will become your place of employment for these few weeks, or longer for those who have chosen to stay home with their babies from now on. If you were at work, you would get a lunch break and a coffee break—take them now.

- Rent some funny movies for your VCR. Now that your social life will be altered a bit, you can bring the movies to you. Make popcorn, set up the movie, sit down with your partner (the baby may even want to sit with you both) and have a "movie night."

- Follow the hints below to prevent frazzled emotions.

  —It is important to find a friend who will allow you to share your feelings and not criticize, personalize, or negate. Your feelings are important! All too often, new parents feel like those around them are judging their parenting skills or competing with them. No one can know how you feel unless you tell them. Remember, you are learning a new role, and there are no rules.
  —If you feel like crying, cry. Crying is an emotional release that can be good for the soul. Think of times when you

cried really hard in times past. How did you feel? Did you feel as though you could sleep for a week? Did the tension disappear from your neck and shoulders? Crying does not only mean that someone is experiencing pain, frustration, anger, and sadness. It may also be a response to joy, happiness, exhaustion, and emotional tension.

If you feel uncomfortable with crying, get in the shower and let the soap get in your eyes...then cry. It is acceptable to cry if you get soap in your eyes!

—Find a new mothers' group. Your childbirth educator or hospital may be able to help you locate one. Many hospitals are beginning to provide postpartum "drop in" groups in response to the shortened hospital stay after delivery. It is important for you to know that you are not alone with your new and at times confusing feelings.

—Put the baby in the carriage or front pack and go for a walk! Babies enjoy fresh air, and so will you. Walking is good exercise and will help you get back in shape. If the weather is bad, get in the car and go to the mall! Many malls are enclosed and are open from early morning until late evening. You will always find people in the mall, and they are often other mothers, fathers, and grandparents. You don't have to shop—you can sit on a bench, get a cold drink, and watch the people.

• Above all, remember that it took about forty weeks for this baby to be ready for birth, and it will take you at least nine months to feel recovered physically and emotionally. Be careful that you don't expect too much from yourself, your partner, and your baby. We all have to *learn* how to be parents. Many women begin to solidify their maternal identity when their baby says "ma-ma." Unfortunately, in our society, many women are led to believe that they will flow with maternal hormones the first time they see their baby. How can you love someone you don't even know?

• There are support groups for new mothers:
Depression After Delivery Support Groups: These groups are growing nationally. They are self-help support groups for women who are experiencing anxiety, depression, and other emotional adjustments to becoming mothers. For information regarding the groups in your area, contact: Depression After Delivery, P.O. Box 1282, Morrisville, Pennsylvania, 19067 (215) 295-3994.

Chapter Ten

For Fathers Only

Now let's talk to fathers only. Yes, fathers, you deserve your own section in this book! It has been quite an experience so far, hasn't it? You have watched, coached, supported, and helped your partner through the labor and delivery of your baby. At times, you may have wanted to run and hide.

Having a baby is an emotionally exhausting experience. You've made all the phone calls, gone to work, rushed home to care for the animals, and then rushed to the hospital to spend time with the new mother and your baby. When you drove the baby home from the hospital the ride may have been the longest on record, as you probably took all the back roads to avoid traffic, or if you live in the city, to avoid the potholes in the roads! After you arrived home you both fell into bed exhausted. Are you having fun yet?

Many times you may have wondered why you haven't received any presents. Maybe you feel as though you have taken a back seat to your baby during these early days. Please remember, *you* are a major player in this new lifestyle called becoming a parent.

Many new fathers have shared with us that it really helps to take a few days off from work after your partner and the baby come home from the hospital. This way the two of you can spend time sharing your thoughts, feelings, and intimacies. It is hard to do that sort of emotional work in the hospital where there are many interruptions and visitors. It also helps, if you are at home, to be the controller of the "at home" visitors. One recommendation is that you stay in your pajamas and lock up the house, pull the drapes, turn on the telephone answering machine, and have a "pajama party." You and your partner are probably just beginning to realize that this baby is yours, as well as beginning to get in touch with the feelings, fears, and concerns of being a "good enough" parent. This "pajama party" will give you time to do this. You will be fine, and you will be good enough. Trust yourself and have faith in your common sense.

Spend time with your baby. One suggestion is to take off your shirt or pajama top and place the baby on your chest, with his head nestled under your chin. It feels wonderful. This is a time to attach to this child and to claim him as yours. It may be a wise idea, if possible, to ask both your parents and hers to stay away for a few days so that the two of you can gain some confidence in your parenting skills. It would be nice to feel that you have begun to master fatherhood before the grandparents (also known as the "experts") arrive.

During your time at home, you will be the chief cook and bottle washer. Your mate needs to physically and emotionally recover, and she really needs your help to do this. Bring her meals in bed and encourage her to sleep when the baby sleeps. If possible, you can nap at this time too. Babies don't sleep for long periods through the night, so you probably won't either. If you can provide for your mate's needs during these early days, you will both benefit.

When your parents do arrive, give them things to do so that they feel as though they are contributing. You may think of your parents a bit differently now, as you start to experience feelings for your tiny baby. They may be acting a bit funny, because they are beginning to reminisce about the days they brought you home from the hospital. They are beginning to think about their new role as grandparents, so in many ways you are all having many new feelings and thoughts. It would be fun to sit around and listen while they share their memories.

After a few weeks you will return to work and will feel as though things are really great. Then comes the three- to six-week "crazies." This is the time when the baby is a bit irritable and decides to be fussy in the early evening, and you may begin to wonder about the whole idea of parenting. Many fathers have shared their feelings about this stage of the postpartum period.

The common scenario is this: you come home from work, exhausted and seeking solace and anxious to see your baby and wife. She is standing at the door holding the baby and waiting for you. She doesn't look very happy. You come up the steps smiling, and she hands the baby to you and tells you she is leaving—the baby has been crying since 2 p.m. and she has had it! For a moment, you may wonder what happened to the capable person that you married. She is like a raving maniac!

Welcome to the postpartum stage. Your fantasy of what the first month with the baby would be like is over, and this is real life! You are now left at the doorway with the baby and you begin to wonder if you should take up jogging, become a couch potato, or perhaps stay at work. Slow down. Let's look closely at your wife's feelings and how normal they are.

At about three to six weeks of age, all babies begin to cry a lot, and begin to experience gas and demonstrate irritable behaviors. This is normal. Also at this time, the women you live with is feeling that she should have things more "in control," and she feels insecure and exhausted. She does not know what you are thinking, but she thinks that you are lucky to be at work and around adults all day. You are thinking how nice it would be to stay home all day with the baby. And because of the craziness of these first few weeks, you may both be so focused on the baby that you have stopped talking with each other. Stop! It is time to get together and share your feelings.

First of all, get a baby swing and put it together. Baby swings are great—most couples are able to sit down and eat dinner with baby swinging in the room. Call the Chinese restaurant and order dinner (and have it delivered!). Now, sit down, relax, and discuss your feelings and concerns about the changes going on in your life. Are you feeling insecure and exhausted, and concerned about being the best dad and husband in the world? Well, she feels the same way. Neither of you will be able to make this baby happy twenty-four hours a day. Can you do that for yourself? So what makes you think that you have that much power over another person, such as your daughter or son? Your children have their own feelings and will share them with you. You will learn to separate your feelings and ideas from those of your children, and will allow them to express their ideas and

Infant Carriers

Front pack carriers are handy for carrying new babies. They allow close, soothing contact, but leave Mom's or Dad's hands free for other activities. As baby develops more head control and gets heavier, he can be carried in a back pack carrier just about anywhere.

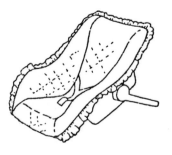

Front pack carrier

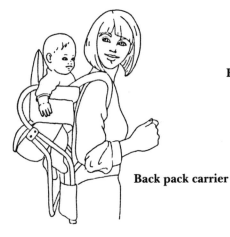

Back pack carrier

Infant seats are convenient when Mom needs her hands free but wants to keep baby in the room with her. They can be placed on the floor or a secure tabletop. Make sure you get one that is made of sturdy materials.

Infant seat

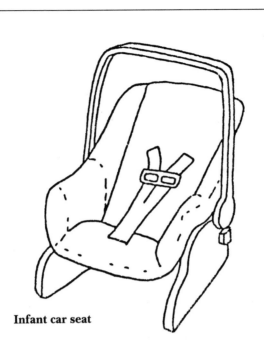

Infant car seat

All infants and children must be safely secured in a moving car. Baby's first trip home from the hospital will be in a car seat—an adult cannot protect an infant-in-arms in a collision. A car seat is used until a child is big or heavy enough to use an adult seat belt. When purchasing an infant car seat, choose one that has been dynamically crash tested and meets federal standards for infant car seats.

The infant seat should be placed facing the back of the car until the baby can sit up by himself. An infant must be properly secured in the shoulder restraints that come with the car seat. *Read the directions* so you know how to do this. Do not put baby in the seat, secure the adult seat belt, and think that this is enough—it isn't! Never use a baby seat, car bed, or any other carrier in a car, even if you put it on the floor or in the back of a station wagon.

Read the pamphlet that comes with your car seat to find out how heavy a child the seat is constructed to hold. Many infant car seats can be used for both infants and toddlers and come with instructions on how to convert the seat for the bigger child.

opinions. You will do the best that you can. You are not perfect; your mate is not perfect; and your child is not perfect.

Rearrange your priorities and develop flexibility and the ability to "go with the flow." This is what parenthood is all about—learning to live with the separate, unique individuals that are our children.

Now, what about each other? Remember, if the two of you feel that your needs are not being met, or if you are drained and emotionally depleted, how can you give to another person? When you feel this way it becomes very hard to be understanding and calm. Maybe you have been at work all day and are exhausted from hearing other peoples' problems, dilemmas, deadlines, etc. You are anxious to go home, sit down, and have some time where no one requires a thing from you. She, on the other hand, has probably been working at home all day and has been, perhaps, literally sucked on all day, while trying to get dinner, do the wash, and tend to the baby. She figures that when you come home, you will take the baby while she takes a shower (she hasn't had time to do that yet!). Instead of being aware of each other's needs at this time, you may each be thinking only of your own needs. This is not uncommon, and is understandable, but it does not make for a happy homecoming!

One big suggestion: talk together and arrange for the Master Plan. This involves "time out" for each of you, but in an orderly way, one that takes the feelings of each of you into account. The plan is this: when you come home from work, you will have a half-hour to do whatever you want. Read the paper, take a shower, sit in a chair and do nothing. Don't talk to each other—just nod. Then, she will give you the baby, and now she has a half-hour to do whatever she wants—take a shower, nap, read a magazine, or sit and meditate. At the end of this total hour, you will greet each other and begin your night at home. Does that sound fair? It has worked successfully for other couples for years. What you end up with is a special time, after work, where you both regroup. As the baby gets older, she may even play quietly while the two of you talk about your day and become friends again. It is impossible to switch hats from one job to the next without taking some time in between. Think about it.

It is important for you to know that you need to learn how to father, she needs to learn how to mother, and collectively you have to learn how to parent. You each bring very unique styles into this relationship. Much of your parenting style depends on how you were raised. Many couples have recommended that each parent have separate times with the baby to accomplish this learning. If the mother, your partner, is always in the room, she will give you suggestions that work for her; if you are alone, you will learn what works for you. Babies are very smart. They know which parent to go to and for what...don't you remember?

Fortunately, these days fathers are getting much-deserved attention. You play a vital role in your child's development. Learn to change your baby's diaper, calm him, and rock him, and find time to spend quiet moments together. Some fathers have found that it is especially nice to take the baby with them in the bathtub. The water is calming and warm, and it is a fun experience. If your partner is breastfeeding, you can carry the baby to her, and when the nursing session is over, take the baby back and cuddle together. After the breastfeeding routine has been well established, some couples will have a bottle feeding (with pumped breast milk) that is "time for Dad." This will have to be discussed. Decide what will be best for you. Feeding isn't the only time you can spend with baby: make other times special for the two of you, too.

Remember that you need to develop your role as a father to your baby, but don't forget to nourish your role as a husband, lover, and friend to your partner.

Chapter Eleven

Is There Sex After Baby?

It is not uncommon for couples to think "There is no rush...I don't really care if we ever have sex again." Many of these thoughts arise from the experience of birth. The woman cannot imagine the thought of the penis near the episiotomy, while the man is wondering if sex will ever be the same after he watched the baby's head stretch the vagina. If she experienced a Cesarean delivery, the mother is afraid of the pressure of her lover on her abdomen during intercourse, and she wonders if they would do better standing up. Other couples have overwhelming sexual feelings for each other after the birth, and are anxious to make love as soon as possible.

Human dynamics are complex, and no two people can feel the same thing. But what about sex? Will you ever make love again? Sexual relations are an intimate form of communication. Sexuality is a part of human dynamics, and sexual needs are important for every couple. So what will you do?

To start, communicate on a verbal level. You are both carrying around fears and fantasies that need to be discussed. The first thing most couples do is collect the concrete facts. When can we physiologically have sex, and what about birth control? These questions require intellectual answers that are easy to obtain. The how-to's require more discussion. So let us first start with the facts.

Many health professionals recommend that sexual intercourse be avoided until the vaginal discharge (lochia) has subsided. This generally happens in two to three weeks. Others will recommend that the woman have her postpartum check for

physiological healing prior to resuming intercourse. Both suggestions are fine—you have to decide collectively which is best
for you.

With regard to contraception: if the woman is breastfeeding,
you need to be cautioned that breastfeeding is *not* a sure-fire
method of contraception. There are no guarantees. In fact, it is
not recommended as a method of contraception, especially in
today's society where babies suck on pacifiers, have relief formula bottles, and are not always fed on a total demand breastfeeding schedule. We have seen too many women have their
second baby within eleven months to put much faith in it at all.
Barrier methods are the recommended contraceptive methods
until the health care professional has been seen for contraceptive counseling after the birth. The condom is the safest and
most reliable method after birth. Many couples have recommended the use of lubricated condoms, as the woman's vaginal
secretions are a bit diminished for a time because of the hormonal changes that take place during the postpartum period. See
the inset on page 143 for a summary of contraceptive methods.

If you use a diaphragm, it will need to be refitted after the
birth, as the cervix size may have changed. The birth control pill
can be prescribed by the health care provider at the six-week
checkup, if indicated.

So now that you have the facts, what are you going to do?
Primarily, the two of you will need to spend some time talking
about your fears related to resuming intercourse. A good way to
begin to get in touch with each other again is to go to bed a little
early—and not to go to sleep. You might start by just hugging,
then move on to kissing, mutual masturbation and pleasuring
techniques, and then finally, at some day or time, having intercourse. There are some important psychosocial issues to take
into account first.

One issue is *body image*. This is how you feel about your body.
How *do* you feel about your body after the birth? Are you concerned about your partner's reaction to your sagging belly, full
breasts, and stretch marks? This is not uncommon. Guys, do you
feel as though she looks fine and are not expecting any problems? Well, talk to each other. Many couples will tell you that the
problems they had were not related to desire; rather, they had
more to do with environment. Just as the two of you are becom-

Methods of Contraception

Barrier Methods

Foam and Condom. This combination is nearly 100 percent effective. The condom prevents sperm from entering the vagina during intercourse, and the spermicidal foam kills sperm. The condom used alone and correctly is about 97 percent effective. The condom provides protection against sexually transmitted diseases.

Diaphragm with Spermicidal Jelly or Cream. The diaphragm is a rubber cup that fits inside the vagina, preventing sperm from entering. The jelly or cream kills the sperm. This method is about 97 percent effective if used correctly.

Vaginal Sponge. This soft, round sponge contains spermicide and is placed inside the vagina, where it both blocks and kills sperm. It is about 89 percent effective.

Cervical Cap. This is another barrier-type device that is filled with spermicide and placed over the cervix. It is about 97 percent effective if used correctly.

Other Methods

Spermicidal Jellies, Foams, and Creams. These kill sperm. Some women say they are inconvenient, messy, and irritate the vagina and penis. They are 90 to 97 percent effective if used correctly.

Intrauterine Device (IUD). The IUD is a small device made of plastic or copper that is placed in the uterus by a doctor. It is about 95 to 99 percent effective, but with its use comes the risk of uterine perforation.

The Pill. The pill is not the best form of contraception for breastfeeding mothers, but it can be appropriate in the lowest effective dose. Progesterone-only preparations show no definite changes in breast milk. There are no reports of adverse effects on infants whose mothers use low-dose pills. The pill is about 99 percent effective if used correctly.

Natural Family Planning. There are several methods in this category. Some involve taking the woman's temperature, checking vaginal secretions, and keeping a careful record of menstrual periods to predict days when she will be fertile. Some of these methods are 90 to 97 percent effective.

Sterilization. Vasectomy for the male, tubal ligation for the female. Sterilization is about 100 percent effective.

ing comfortable and turned on, don't be surprised if the baby begins to stir! That's the end of that!

What if the baby is in your room? Have you thought of moving the bassinet out for a while? Maybe you could put it in another room.

Lets talk about some practical aspects of resuming sexual intercourse. In the list below we have pointed out some aspects of resuming a sexual relationship that concern most new parents.

- Resume intercourse whenever you both are ready.
- Where should you do it? If the baby is in your room, you may find that it is useful to move the bassinet to another room for a time. Although this is not mandatory, it may keep interruptions to a minimum.
- You will have to find a comfortable position for sex. If the woman had an episiotomy, she may find that the most comfortable position, in the beginning, is for her to be in the superior position (on the top). This way, she can control the amount of pressure of the penile shaft near the episiotomy scar. This is also a good position for the woman who has had a Cesarean birth as there is no pressure on her belly.
- Some women complain of vaginal dryness after birth as a result of hormonal changes. Mothers who breastfeed especially have this problem. One way to manage this temporary condition is to use a water-soluble lubricant such as KY jelly. Petroleum-based products are not recommended for this purpose. Many couples have shared that digital foreplay has helped facilitate lubrication of the vagina.
- Breast stimulation is an issue if you are breastfeeding. We are often asked whether breast stimulation is a good idea if the mother is nursing. The father may wonder what will happen if he stimulates her breasts or plays with the nipples. The important point to remember is that if it feels good, why not? Most probably, the milk will "let down" in response to the tactile stimulation. If the woman experiences an orgasm, the milk will begin to flow. This is caused by the secretion of the hormone oxytocin, which is involved in both orgasm and breast milk ejection. If either of you are uncomfortable with this potential response, the woman may

try nursing the baby prior to making love, or wear a bra. Some men have suggested that you just have a towel ready!
- The most important thing to remember is to keep your sense of humor, relax, and enjoy each other.

Many couples have found that they experience a change in their sexuality after childbearing. Is it because you feel closer to each other as a result of the love you feel for your child? Is it the increased trust in your relationship as a result of the shared birth? Or does it have to do with the fact that the woman may feel more in touch with her sexuality as a result of childbearing? Based on the uniqueness of human relations, there is no right answer. How does it feel for you?

A word about orgasms. It is normal not to experience orgasm the first time you have sex after the birth. In fact, it may take time. This could be because you may both be a bit nervous the first few times and will not really relax and enjoy yourselves. The important thing is to talk about what feels good and to share intimacies with each other.

So yes, there is sex after babies. It is just different for a while. It is important to remember to start out verbally communicating your feelings. Soon, you will be showing your love for each other physically, too.

As you grow and develop as parents, please take time to assess how far you have come. Your baby needs you both to be in touch with your feelings. He also needs the security that your relationship will provide for him.

This new job you have undertaken is filled with every emotion imaginable. It is a lot of work, but most of us cannot think of a more exciting career.

Chapter Twelve

Roles and Relationships

GRANDPARENTS (YOUR PARENTS)

Let's talk about the other people in your life. First, your parents. On one hand, you want your mother to comfort you, but on the other hand, as a capable young woman who has just given birth, you resent her interventions and suggestions. This is all very normal. If you put it into perspective, you will become aware that your parents—and his parents—also have to adjust to your baby's birth. They are now grandparents!

The media often portrays grandparents as aged, gray, fragile people. The reality of today is that grandparents are dynamic, active, and involved men and women. In many cases, they may not even have time to see you until the weekend because of their careers, or because they do not live in the same state.

Your mother has probably relived your birth through your experience, and she may have her own issues to resolve. In her day, the baby's father was rarely in attendance during the birth. Nor did they have disposable diapers or ready-made formula available to them, and breastfeeding was discouraged. So your mother watches you with mixed emotions. She may be mourning her own roles—she is your mother, but now she is also a grandmother. She now has to re-evaluate her role as a parent. Your Dad may be quietly standing on the side, reminiscing about the day when he held you for the first time. You see, it is through our children, in many ways, that we become "grown up." And as many mothers will tell you, this job never ends, even when our children grow up and have children of their own.

Your parents want the best for you, and at the same time, they are acutely aware of some of both the sorrows and joys of parenthood.

The relationship of new mothers and fathers to their parents may be a source of some conflict during these early weeks of parenthood. It is important to discuss issues, feelings, and concerns, and to share wonderment as well as sadness. It is by becoming parents that many of us will begin to acknowledge our parents as people. You will wonder how they managed with five children! You may gain a new sense of respect for them. But you will definitely come to realize that they were never perfect, and probably never tried to be. You will understand that they did the best they could do with the situations that confronted them, and that is really all you can do, too.

Grandparents can give your baby a special love that is all-encompassing. They do not have to set limits—that is your job now. So let them have a good time, keep clear as to who is in charge of this baby, and keep communication open. You cannot spoil a new baby with too much love and attention.

FRIENDS AND ACQUAINTANCES

What about friends? Do you have any friends with children? Or when you were without children, did you avoid interacting with these people, because all they did was talk about their babies? Interestingly enough, you now know why they carried fifty snapshots of their baby for the world to see, and why they spoke with such pride when their baby slept through the night for the first time. Go and renew your relationships with these people! They can give you a lot of support, especially if they are honest and willing to share with you some of the concerns they had when they were learning to become parents.

What if you are the first in your group to have a baby? Then it is imperative that you join a new parents group or go to a postpartum exercise class to make new friends. You will find that having a baby will help you initiate relationships with people that you would have never spoken to before. We all like to talk about our children.

The mall is a great place to go during the day. You can push your baby in the stroller and stop and sit on a bench and talk to other mothers and fathers who are "hanging out" there. This is an especially good place to go in bad weather, because you can be out of the house and get some exercise and see people.

VISITORS

Let's talk about these people again. You will find that visitors are a major problem during the early weeks after the birth. After that their visits become less frequent. Your real friends may have delivered meals to your door, helped clean your house, or taken your other children (if there are any) out to the park. It is the visitors who arrive to see the baby and who want to be entertained that you need to be cautious of.

One technique that worked well for one lady was to keep an old housecoat by the door. When the doorbell rang, she would put the coat on and slowly open the door, appearing as if she had just gotten out of bed. Her friends would look at her and tell her that since she looked so tired, they would not stay, but that they wanted to drop off the present and would call again in a few weeks. She would thank them, close the door, take off the robe, and go on with her activities.

Another father suggested that he would play the heavy and limit the visits to about ten minutes, then ask the person to come at another time. Your mother or his mother can also take care of this for you. "My daughter (in-law) needs to rest now, so could you please come back at another time?" works wonders.

You may find that when the house is full of company, the only way to escape is to take the baby into your bedroom and feed him. If you are breastfeeding, you will probably not have the confidence to nurse discreetly with an audience, so protect yourself. You can also fall asleep with the baby in your own room and never have to come out until you wake up and they are all gone. These are some suggestions.

Be aware that in many ways you may want to socialize with your visitors, but it requires emotional energy, and you may not have much of that during the early days. Also remember that most of the visitors will go home and be able to sleep through the night—that is a privilege you will not experience for some time.

YOUR RELATIONSHIP TO YOUR MATE

The relationship between the new mother and new father is important. You have both experienced an unbelievable and emotional time. You will now need to work on expanding your relationship to include another person. A couple's relationship needs to be nurtured. Communication and focused time are important.

Have you had time to talk with each other about what the birth was like? Have you had time to just hold each other and watch your baby sleeping in the bassinet? Or do you feel as though you are both living in different places at the same time?

Communication is imperative. You cannot read each others' minds, and must avoid assuming feelings and behaviors. If this is your first baby, neither one of you probably feels like an expert. You may each bring to this experience preconceived ideas and feelings that have no basis. It is not uncommon to hear couples talk about competitive parenting. That is when they are at odds as to who gets to do what, and do not acknowledge that they each have a unique role as well as a collaborative role. Let us take some time to discuss this issue.

Each of you bring into this new role experiences and expectations from your past. You also have fantasies about how you will perform as parents. It is important to talk about these ideas so that you decide how you will manage with your baby and yourselves as parents. You may be wondering how you will ever even get to be in the same room at the same time to talk at all, but you will if you take the time. You have to plan it. After babies, you may tend to take each other for granted and then end up exchanging evil looks as you pass. This is not healthy. Nor is it uncommon. The following are some ways you can make your relationship a priority.

- Go to bed early and at the same time ... you do not have to go to sleep! Now you can look at each other and stare. After a while you may even talk. As you progress, you may hug and then even kiss. ... (See Chapter Eleven for more about this.)
- Make appointments for tea or coffee together. Depending on work schedules, this may be in the morning or in the evening after the children are in bed.
- Court each other. Leave notes in his lunch box, send her cards through the mail—do something nice for each other.

- Go out on a date. Remember dates? Avoid going to the movies because you will not talk to each other during that two hours! How about going for a walk around the block? You can even do this with the baby in a front carrier. Hold hands and laugh out loud (remember how good that used to feel?).
- You may wonder where you will find a babysitter you can trust. Are your parents around? They would love to watch the baby for a few hours. What about friends with children? How about swapping babies and time? Call your community service programs and see if they conduct babysitting courses and secure names that way. Talk with your neighbors—who do they use? Many times your single friends would love to watch a baby for a few hours. Some of them think it is fun!

Remember that the two of you started out together and hope to remain together as your child gets older...nourish that relationship.

The key factor is emotional availability. If you do not take good care of each other, you will not have a whole lot left over to give to your daughter or son.

Well, how are you feeling now? We hope that you feel more confident as you live together as new parents. We have attempted to provide you with reality-based information and suggestions about this life. Our hope is that you will come to trust your intuitions and feel competent in this new job. *You* are the experts.

Parenthood is a full-time profession. It requires commitment, support, humor, and most of all, common sense. Trust yourselves and have fun.

Recommended Reading

Barbach, L. *For Each Other: Sharing Sexual Intimacy*. New York: Doubleday, 1982.

Barber, Virginia, and Merrill Maguire Skaggs. *The Mother Person*. New York: Bobbs-Merrill, 1977.

Brazelton, T. Berry. *On Becoming a Family: The Growth of Attachment*. New York: Delacorte Press, 1981.

Cole, K. C. *What Only a Mother Can Tell You About Having a Baby*. New York: Berkley Books, 1980.

Comfort, A. *The Joy of Sex*. New York: Simon and Schuster, 1974.

Dix, Carol. *The New Mother Syndrome*. New York: Pocket Books, 1985.

Dodson, Fitzhugh. *How to Father*. Los Angeles: Nash, 1974.

Eagan, Andrea Boroff. *The Newborn Mother: Stages of Growth*. Boston: Little, Brown & Company, 1985.

Galinsky, Ellen. *Between Generations: The Stages of Parenthood*. New York: Berkley Books, 1981.

Genevie, Louis, and Eva Margolies. *The Motherhood Report: How Women Feel About Being Mothers*. New York: Macmillan, 1987.

Grams, Marilyn. *Breastfeeding Source Book*. Sheridan, Wyoming: Achievement Press, 1988.

Gresh, Sean. *Becoming a Father*. New York: Butterick Publishers, 1980.

Harris, Robie H. and Elizabeth Levy. *Before You Were Three: How You Began to Walk, Talk, Explore and Have Feelings.* New York: Delacorte Press, 1977.

Heffner, Elaine. *Mothering: The Emotional Experience of Mothering After Freud and Feminism.* New York: Doubleday and Company, 1978.

Huggins, Kathleen. *Nursing Mothers' Companion.* Boston: Harvard Common Press, 1986.

Jones, Sandy. *Crying Babies, Sleepless Nights.* New York: Warner Books, 1983.

Kelly, Marguerite and Elia Parsons. *Mother's Almanac.* Garden City, New York: Doubleday, 1975.

Kitzinger, Sheila. *Women's Experience of Sex.* New York: Penguin Books, 1983.

Kort, Carol and Ronnie Friedland. *The Mothers' Book: Shared Experiences.* New York: Houghton Mifflin, 1981.

Kort, Carol and Ronnie Friedland. *The Fathers' Book: Shared Experiences.* New York: Houghton Mifflin, 1986.

Lazarre, Jane. *The Mother Knot.* New York: McGraw-Hill, 1976.

Leach, Penelope. *The First Six Months: Getting Together With Your Baby.* New York: Alfred A. Knopf, 1987.

Leach, Penelope. *Your Baby and Child From Birth to Age Five.* New York: Alfred A. Knopf, 1978.

Lesko, Wendy, and Matthew M. Lesko. *The Maternity Sourcebook.* New York: Warner Books, 1985.

Linden, Paula and Susan Gross. *Taking Care of Mommy.* Garden City, New York: Doubleday, 1983.

Norris, Gloria and JoAnn J. Miller. *The Working Mother's Complete Handbook.* New York: New American Library, 1984.

Olds, Sally Wendkos. *The Working Parent's Survival Guide.* New York: Bantam Books, 1983.

Piljac, Pamela. *You Can Go Home Again: The Career Woman's Guide to Leaving the Work Force.* Portage, Indiana: Bryce-Waterton Publishers, 1985.

Rakowitz, Elly and Gloria S. Rubin. *Living With Your New Baby.* New York: Berkley Books, 1978.

Rich, Adrienne. *Of Woman Born: Motherhood as Experience and Institution.* New York: W.W. Norton and Company, 1976.

Satter, Ellyn. *Child of Mine: Feeding With Love and Good Sense.* Palo Alto, California: Bull Publishing Company, 1986.

Shield, Renee Rose. *Making Babies in the '80s: Common Sense for New Parents*. Boston: Harvard Common Press, 1983.

Winnicott, D.W. *Babies and Their Mothers*. Reading, Massachusetts: Addison-Wesley Publishing Company, 1987.

Winnicott, D.W. *The Child, the Family and the Outside World*. Reading Massachusetts: Addison-Wesley Publishing, 1987.

Yaffe, Maurice and Elizabeth Fenwick. *Sexual Happiness: A Practical Approach*. New York: Henry Holt and Company, 1988.

Video:

Diapers and Delirium: The Care and Comfort of Parents of Newborns. This video is available for $24.95 plus $3.00 shipping and handling from Lifecycle Productions, Inc., P.O. Box 183, Newton, MA 02165, or call 1-800-242-1520.

In this lively video Jeanne Watson Driscoll discusses coping with living with your new baby. You'll laugh and cry as other parents share their experiences, and you'll learn that you're not alone!

About the Authors

Jeanne Watson Driscoll, MS, RN, CS, IBCLC: Jeanne Driscoll is the partner and cofounder of Lactation Associates and vice president and cofounder of Lifecycle Productions, Inc. in Waltham, Massachusetts.

She is also in private practice as a nurse psychotherapist specializing in Postpartum Psychiatric Disorders in association with Dr. Deborah Sichel. Jeanne was formally associated with Brigham and Womens' Hospital in Boston, Massachusetts as the Mental Health Clinical Nurse Specialist and Lactation Consultant.

Jeanne is a nationally known speaker on issues of breastfeeding management as well as psychosocial aspects of pregnancy and postpartum. Her works have appeared in both lay and professional journals. Jeanne is a member of the American Nurses' Association, Massachusetts Nurses' Association, Sigma Theta Tau (National Honor Society of Nurses), The International Lactation Consultants' Association, and the International Childbirth Education Association.

Marsha Walker, RN, BS, BA, ACCE, IBCLC: Marsha Walker is the partner and cofounder of Lactation Associates. She is also the director of the Breastfeeding Support Program at Harvard Community Health Plan in Wellesley, Massachusetts.

Marsha is a nationally known speaker on issues of breastfeeding management and has had articles published in both professional and lay journals. She is a member of The American Nurses' Association, Massachusetts Nurses' Association, Sigma Theta Tau, American Society of Psychoprophylaxis in Obstetrics, International Lactation Consultants' Association, and The International Childbirth Education Association.

Index